The Pocket
POWTER

**Questions and Answers
to Help You Change the Way
You Look and Feel Forever**

Susan Powter ™

A FIRESIDE BOOK
Published by Simon & Schuster
New York London Toronto Sydney Tokyo Singapore

FIRESIDE
Rockefeller Center
1230 Avenue of the Americas
New York, New York 10020

FIRESIDE and colophon are registered trademarks
of Simon & Schuster Inc.
Designed by Bonni Leon
Manufactured in the United States of America

10 9 8 7 6 5 4 3 2 1

Library of Congress Cataloging-in-Publication Data
Powter, Susan, date.
The pocket Powter : questions and answers to help you
change the way you look and feel forever / Susan Powter.
p. cm.
"A Fireside book."
1. Reducing. 2. Women—Nutrition. 3. Exercise for women.
4. Physical fitness for women. I. Title.
RA778.P8835   1994
613.7'045—dc20   94-4648
CIP

ISBN: 0-671-89456-0

CONTENTS

Introduction   7

Eat   11
*"You can get lean, but you must start with eating.
Guess what? Food doesn't make you fat—
fat makes you fat."*

Breathe   109
*"Oxygen equals energy. Get back into the habit
of breathing, learn to do it correctly, and
take a few lifesaving breaths each day."*

Move   123
*"It's time to use movement to change your body.
It's easy—burn some fat, increase some strength."*

Live   197
*"Get your life back, and gain strength, choices, and
power that you've never had."*

You Ask, I Answer . . .   237
*"If you want to know about me, don't read
the tabloids. Ask me!"*

INTRODUCTION

There isn't any one who doesn't want to look and feel good. We may all have different definitions of what looking and feeling good is, but there's one thing that's the same for all of us—the way to get there.

If you want to be lean, strong, and healthy, to be physically fit and wake up every day with the energy and strength you want to live your life, then there's only one way to do it. You gotta eat, you gotta breathe, and you gotta move.

Within your fitness level, physical considerations, lifestyle, and budget so you can get as lean, as strong, and as healthy as you want to be.

Easy. Done. But what we've been doing so far hasn't worked. Stopping the Insanity is different, and since it's different, there are bound to be questions along the way.

That, my friends, is where *The Pocket Powter* comes in.

Have no fear, the women of America are here. *The Pocket Powter* is the answer to your questions about food, movement, and oxygen. After reading *Stop the Insanity!* thousands of women sent me comments, quotes, suggestions, and questions about changing the way they look and feel forever. *The Pocket Powter* is about the networking and supporting that we need to do to get this informa-

INTRODUCTION

tion to as many people as possible—and that's why
I wrote it.

For you.

So that your transition from a high-fat, unfit, unhealthy lifestyle to a lean, healthy, energy-filled
life is as easy as it can be—and so that we can
share our questions, concerns, fears, joys, suc-
cesses, and goals.

Even though we've got to do the same thing to get
there, our considerations are different. My experiences may not be what you need to apply this information to your life, but I'll guarantee you there is
someone's story out there that will touch your soul,
someone's helpful tip that will answer your question, and someone's pain and resolution that will
help you face your own.

I lost 133 pounds, but I didn't go from a fat person to
a skinny person—I went from an unfit person to a
very fit person, and so can you.

Skinny is out, gone forever. Fit is in, and is a heck
of a lot easier to get than skinny.

Going from 43% body fat to 14% body fat, regaining cardio-endurance that I thought I'd never have,
increasing muscle mass and strength beyond my
wildest dreams, and regaining control of my life was
a matter of getting and learning to apply the right
information.

INTRODUCTION

Fortunately, this is no longer my story. This is the story of the hundreds of thousands of women who are never dieting again—eating more than they ever dreamed possible, moving within their fitness level, regaining the energy that had been long gone in their lives, and getting well. ... A wonderful side effect of getting well is loving the way you look and feel: regaining your body, seeing muscles for the first time in years, and watching the dress sizes plummet—that's big fun, you'll see!

So we all kind of wrote this *Pocket Powter* together, so you could get the information you need to reach your fitness goal.

Do me a favor. Send me your comments, your favorite reduced-fat recipes, tips, questions, or anything else you want to send, because there are going to be more Powters coming (not kids, I've got my hands full there—but *Pocket Powter 2, 4, 10, 16*—just like the movie sequels, these may keep on coming and never die). In the back of your *Pocket Powter* are my address and phone number. Talk to me.

Share and network with us, because hating the way we look and feel, not having the energy to get through the day, and being physically unwell is a problem that affects millions of us. Let's stop treat-

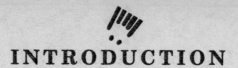

INTRODUCTION

ing the symptoms—and start solving the problem together.

Health and happiness to you.

Be well,

Susan Powter™

Susan Powter

EAT

*You don't have to be afraid
of food anymore.*

EAT

Eating.

I know, I know, it scares the hell out of you, doesn't it?

Eat means fat. Fat means feeling awful, and being fat means dieting. Starvation, deprivation, and dying of hunger. Eating, binging, and dieting again. The Catch-22.

Well, not anymore.

Diets don't work. You and I know that, because between us we've tried every diet under the sun.

Has it worked so far? Do you love the way you look? Thighs just like you want them to be?

NO CHANCE. Because there isn't a diet on earth that works.

If there was, there'd be one very rich person living on this planet, and there wouldn't be a fat person around, because nobody likes looking and feeling bad—and it's not as if we haven't tried starving the weight off thousands of times.

Ninety-eight percent of us who lose weight by reducing calories, starving, depriving ourselves—that is, *dieting*—will gain the weight back. Those are the diet industry's stats, not mine, but I'd say they speak for themselves.

Diets don't work, but eating does.

Food doesn't make you fat—fat makes you fat.

Without fuel your body can't function, doesn't have the energy it needs to get through the day, and guess

EAT

what? The first symptom of deprivation is binging.

These topics are just some of what we talked about in *Stop the Insanity!* and some of the issues we'll be taking on in the Eating section of *The Pocket Powter*.

Eating may be hard to get used to because we've been taught not to eat. But the more you know, the more you understand, and the easier it'll be. Take it from me and hundreds of thousands of women who have tried it—eating is a whole lot easier to live with than starvation.

So—let's learn how to eat.

EAT

What does the fat formula tell me? Why do I multiply the fat grams times 9?

The fat formula tells you exactly how much fat is in each serving of food—and it helps you make low-fat choices. The reason you multiply the grams times 9 is because of the inequality of calories:

One gram of carbohydrates equals 4 calories.
One gram of protein equals 4 calories.
One gram of fat equals—no, not 4, not 6 . . .
One gram of fat equals 9 calories.
Fat is fat.

Calories are your fuel. And fat makes you fat.

EAT

How do I figure out what 30% of my daily intake is? Do I have to add up everything I eat for the day?

The old "30% of daily intake" had me confused when I first started changing my body.

Here's how you can figure out your total daily fat intake, whether it's 10% or 30%, and remember—that decision is yours to make based on how much fat you need to lose.

You have a choice.

In the beginning, you can do the fat formula on everything you put into your mouth, and if it reads 30% or less, eat it. You cannot exceed 30% of your daily intake if nothing you put into your mouth is over 30% fat. That's what I did, because it's the easiest way. Very soon you'll not only know where the fat is, but also where it isn't. Those are the foods—and there are tons of them out there—that you'll work with, creating the tastes and textures you love.

There's another way. You can write down everything you eat—the total calories in one column and the fat grams in another—and at the end of the day do the fat formula on the total. I don't know about you, but I don't have the time for that, and besides, writing down everything you eat forces you to keep a food journal, and again—the old diet thinking. Who wants to get into that?

EAT

How do I decide what percentage of fat to eat?

It's been decided for you by a couple of experts. The AMA (American Medical Association) suggests that your daily intake be 30% of your total caloric intake ... but what do they know? The real nutrition and food experts suggest anywhere from 10% to 30%, 30% being the high end. Within that range, *you* decide.

Do you have tons (pardon the pun) of fat to lose? Are you dealing with a heart condition? Then go to the lower daily fat percentages.

Do you want to see results and start to shrink? Then go LOW with the fat, go HIGH with the quality and volume of your food, and MOVE, MOVE, MOVE within your fitness level. You'll be in like Flynn (what *does* that expression mean???).

My body is becoming a fat-burning machine, and soon it will be lean, strong, and healthy.
> —K.K., Ohio

EAT

What about all those fat-free products?

Fat-free—isn't everything fat-free these days? If it isn't fat-free, it's lean, light, and you know there's no cholesterol in it because there's no cholesterol in anything anymore, haven't you noticed?

Well, you and I have to know better because they—the label liars—are trying to scam us all in a big way.

If there is food in it, there is fat in it. The label law loophole that these companies use to get away with that fat-free claim is that if the fat's below a certain percentage per serving, they are allowed to say "fat-free." Fat-free means it's low-fat, but it can also mean that it's loaded with sugar. So, fellow fat detectives, read your labels, question every fat-free claim, and arm yourselves with that fat formula.

Here it is:

Take the number of fat grams per serving × 9 = X.
Take X and divide it by the total number of calories.
That will tell you how much of the serving you are about to eat is fat.

Let's look at a sample label together. It's for a brand of popcorn that screams at us from the label, "one-third less calories, fat, and oil."

EAT

Nutrition Information (per serving)

Serving size	9.5 grams (approx. 1 cup)
Servings per bag	18
Calories	35
Protein	1 g
Carbohydrates	6 g
Fat	2 g
Sodium	85 mg

Popcorn is a low-fat food, so let's do the formula and confirm it.

Two grams of fat—that's pretty low. You should be able to eat as much of this as you want, right? But first check the formula:

2 grams × 9 calories = 18.
18 divided by the total calories of 35 equals what? .51.

That's 51% fat in every serving!

"Fat makes you fat." It sounds so simple. It can be that simple sometimes.
— D.B., Kentucky

EAT

***I've heard about the new nutritional labeling.
Will I still need to do the fat formula?***

OHHHHHHHHHHHHHHHHH. . . . Yes, you still
need the fat formula.

You might not believe this, but not only will you
still be using the fat formula, those new labels cost
us—the taxpayers—somewhere between $1.4 billion
and $2.3 billion!

Yep, you and I will still be doing the formula till
the cows come home, or till the boys in the FDA
(Food and Drug Administration) give us what we
want:

How much fat is in this serving of food? Is it high,
or is it low?

*Ignore the labels, write your Congressperson, and
use your fat formula.*

EAT

Some products don't have nutritional information on the package. How do I know if they're okay to eat?

If it's not labeled—RUN, RUN, RUN for your life!

Food manufacturers get away with murder with all the label loopholes when they are required to put it all down—can you imagine what goes into your food when they are not required to label? HELLLL-LLLLLLLLLLLLLLLLLLLPPPPP me!

If you need to know the fat content of a piece of chicken or something prepackaged, look it up in one of those fat counter guides that you see everywhere. Look up the food in question and you'll see a couple of columns: the calorie column, the fat gram column. . . . Then do your formula. Number of fat grams times 9 equals X. X divided by the total calories will tell you per serving how much fat is in the food you are about to eat.

EAT

I'm so confused. How can a manufacturer say "98% fat-free" when it's not true?

Good question, and one that definitely deserves an answer.

Because all they really care about is getting you to buy their product. They do and will continue to do so as long as we let them get away with it.

The women of America are busting the diet industry, the lying food manufacturers, and the fitness industry. It's time we stopped being the codependent enablers we've been and force them to be responsible to us and our families.

We spend our hard-earned money, we have trusted them, and we deserve the truth. Demand it—you just may start to get a little respect in more ways than one.

Woman, bent upon her freedom and seeking to make a better world, will not permit the forces of reaction to mask themselves forever behind the plea that it is necessary to keep her ignorance to preserve per purity.
                                            —Margaret Sanger

EAT

Do I need to count fat grams?

Not anymore, as Peter Sellers said when he smashed the Steinway piano!

Why?

I mean, after all, who's going to write it down, keep track of it, and figure it all out—

NOT YOU!

You are going to be too busy eating, breathing, and moving to worry about such things.

Doing the fat formula is the easiest, quickest way to figure out the one thing you want to know: How much fat is in this serving of food that I'm about to eat?

The guys who invented this really knew what they were doing. It works, and it's easy.

Well done, boys.

The more you use the fat formula, the easier it is.

EAT

Can I eat too little fat?

Yeah, you can, but it's really hard to do. Most of us don't ever have to worry about eating too little fat. If you eat a wide variety of high-quality food, you'll get the essential fatty acids your body needs to survive. It's not a concern.

And—you don't need to add fat to your diet so that your skin stays moist. . . . I swear, it's something a 300-pound woman told me her doctor told her!

But you do need to worry if you are carrying around excessive body fat, so reduce your body fat percentage to a healthy number and worry about going too low when you get there. . . .

Such a problem. . . . "Oh, no, I'm getting too lean, strong, and healthy, I need to start putting on some bulk." It's a great problem to have—take it from the thousands of women who are experiencing it for the first time!

I've been fit and I've been fat, and fit is better.

EAT

I understand what low-fat is, but what do you mean by high-volume?

Tons of food.

Three squares a day.

Snacks aplenty.

Strong, bulky food.

Strengthening food. Food that lasts—grains, veggies, pastas, fruit, potatoes, beans. . . .

More food than you ever could have dreamed of eating if you want to get lean, be strong, and feel healthy again.

That's it, right there.

Too much of a good thing can be wonderful.
                                    —Mae West

EAT

What do you mean by high-quality food?

A huge plate of sautéed veggies and brown rice with soy lemon sauce, a big piece of fresh cornbread to soak up the juice, and fresh fruit compote with hot strawberry sauce on top for dessert versus a frozen diet dinner.

That's what I had for dinner last night, so I'm using it as the example.

I think frozen diet dinners are crap. My dinner is high-quality, low-fat, loaded with nutrition, high-volume, very filling, and extremely satisfying. . . .

That's eating—and eating is big fun!

EAT

Am I going to have to become a gourmet cook to eat this way?

Gourmet? What's so gourmet about pasta?

Is rice gourmet? Ask your local Chinese restaurant.

Not only do you not need to be a gourmet "anything," you don't need to spend much time in the kitchen because eating high-volume, low-fat food is easy, you can find it anywhere, it's convenient, and it doesn't take much time to prepare.

I think to qualify as a gourmet cook you need to spend more than a couple of hours a week in the kitchen, don't you?

So—we are all off the hook.

EAT

Do I have to eat like this for the rest of my life?

Yeah, why not? Eating a wide variety of high-volume, high-quality, low-fat food—what's the matter with that? You must minimize your daily fat intake, and increase the quality and quantity of what you eat if you want to be lean, strong, and healthy.

OR—you can increase the fat, decrease the quantity—that is, diet—and forget about the quality, and you'll be . . . FAT.

Sure, you have to eat this way for the rest of your life, because for the rest of your life you want to love the way you look and feel and be well—don't you?

The true fact is that inside me is a strong woman. I need to be healthy! Being healthy is not about starvation, or even just losing weight. It's about being healthy.

—T.N., New Jersey

EAT

Susan, what do you eat? I want to eat exactly what you eat.

No—no, you don't, because our tastes and lifestyles are different. You want to eat whatever *you* want, whenever you want it, without getting fat and looking and feeling bad.

I eat different things every day, every hour, every minute that I eat. You want the *freedom* to choose and eat what you want. Believe me, that's a lot better than being dependent on anyone.

Learning how to eat again is as much about getting back in touch with your body and its need for fuel as it is about what kind of fuel you are putting in.

EAT

Can I eat too many calories?

Absolutely. You can eat too many fat calories easily—that's one of the things that makes you fat. And, if you are not moving and are eating thousands of calories, you WILL get fat.

Can you eat too many calories if you are eating high-quality, low-fat calories, moving, and building lean muscle mass? Try it—I haven't found a way to eat too many calories, and I eat like an animal.

This is a question you're not going to worry about when you learn how to eat, how to breathe, and how to move your way to a strong and healthy body.

EAT

Do I need to keep track of my calories if I am watching the fat percentage?

If you don't move, you do.

You can't consume 3,000 calories a day and lie on the sofa and not gain weight.

Eating, breathing, and moving are EQUALLY (*equally* being the operative word here) important. One without the other ain't gonna happen.

Think about it. Without food you don't have the energy to move; without moving you can't burn the fat, increase the metabolism, and get the oxygen; and without the oxygen you'll die!!!!!

They work so beautifully together. This system works.

EÄT

What happens when I eat under 1,000 calories a day?

Nothing, if you are a gerbil, or someone who literally doesn't leave the sofa all day, but if you want to function normally, you won't have enough fuel to function and your body will accommodate by

1. Slowing down its metabolic rate
2. Burning lean muscle mass as fuel—after all, you're not giving it what it needs
3. Craving high-calorie foods—your body is screaming EAT THE DING DONGS, EAT ANYTHING, I'M STARVING!!!
4. Storing the fuel that lasts the longest in famine, because that's what you're in—guess what that fuel is? FAT. That's right, fat.

If you are taking in less than you expend—dieting—eating under 1,000 calories a day, you are going to become weaker and fatter.

Instead of starving, try eating. Take it from me, you'll love it.

The first symptom of starving is binging.

EAT

I have trouble eating this much food. What should I do?

I LOVE THIS. I LOVE THIS A LOT!

Trouble eating this much!

Doesn't that sound a whole lot better than "I'm dying of starvation and can't control my urge to eat"?

This is an easy answer. *Don't eat so much at one sitting.* Eat smaller meals five or six times a day. The amount of calories you take in daily depends on your energy expended and the shape your body's in.

Please don't force-feed. That's just as bad as starvation.

But such a problem, who should worry?

Nothing in life is to be feared, it is only to be understood.

—Marie Curie

EAT

I seem to be hungry a lot. Is it okay to eat when I'm hungry?

That's not just okay . . . . that's brilliant. Congratulations! You are a genius.

This time I know it's different. I love the food I eat. I don't feel deprived and this is how I want to live.
—C.R., Mississippi

EAT

I'm afraid to eat. Food scares me. What can I do?

I understand this fear, and so does every woman in this country who has been on a diet and is afraid of food. You're not alone—millions of us are with you.

Here's what you do:

Get used to eating. Start by eating five or six small meals a day.

Get back into the habit of eating. Isn't it amazing that we have to do this at all? Oh, well, it's time to solve the problem.

Think about what food is—your fuel, your energy, your gasoline.

Learn to eat without fear by eating high-volume, high-quality, low-fat food. You'll never be afraid of food again when you see how lean, strong, and healthy you get by learning how to eat, breathe, and move.

Remember, we're with you.

And the trouble is, if you don't risk anything, you risk even more.

—Erica Jong

EAT

Does it matter when I eat?

Talk about a question that everyone's got an opinion about! Study after study has been done on this question and still—nobody knows for sure. I'll tell you what's more important than *when* you eat: what you eat.

I eat when I'm hungry and sometimes—many times, as a matter of fact—I'm hungry late at night. In my opinion, there's nothing better than a big bowl of cereal while you're watching an old movie late at night in bed with someone you love . . . and remember, that someone you love may just be you. You, the bowl of cereal, and the old movie—heaven, as far as I'm concerned.

It hasn't made a damn bit of difference in my losing 133 pounds and getting well. But don't eat steak at 1:30 A.M. each night—that *will* make a big difference in how you look and feel.

So, can I eat after 7 P.M.?

Sure, if you're hungry and it's high-quality, low-fat fuel, why not? Does the fat wizard fly down and put a spell on your body after 7 P.M.? (If so, I'm in trouble. . . .)

But remember, you gotta move the next day.

EAT

What if I want to eat one large meal instead of several meals throughout the day? Is that okay?

When you start seeing food as fuel, the concept of constant eating makes a whole lot of sense. When you eat during the day, you are feeding your fire—putting the coal in your furnace so you have a nice, strong, hot, consistent flame. Eating one big meal a day is like throwing all your coal into your fire at once. It will burn out, and you won't have the heat/energy/flame that you need to get through the day.

One meal a day would also mean that you'd have to get all your daily calories into one meal. That's a hell of a lot of calories to down at one time.

So, no, don't eat one meal a day. Start with breakfast, lunch, and dinner—that's normal, that's sane. Then, if you're still hungry, eat.

EAT

Is it okay to eat between meals? Sometimes in the afternoon I get really hungry.

Of course you do. You've been running all day, it's probably been hours since lunch, and it's time to chow down.

Whoever said you couldn't eat until 6 P.M.? Probably the same idiot who said everybody should live on 1,000 calories a day, no matter what their activity level!!!!

Yes, take the time, sit and eat and enjoy, because you are going to have a lot more energy to get through the rest of the afternoon, evening, and night if you eat.

It really makes sense to me. And how easy! I thought, "You are telling me to eat. I can do this, I can eat!"

—N.C., Nevada

EAT

I'm a very busy person and I find myself snacking all day instead of really eating meals. Is this okay?

Hi, fellow very busy person—good to meet you!

I absolutely understand this problem, but the answer to your question is NO, NO, NO, it is not okay to snack instead of eat.

Snacking is okay if you've eaten food, a real meal, but substituting a snack for a meal won't get you the quality, the volume, or the low-fat, wide variety of foods you need to change the way you look and feel.

How about doing what I do, and snack on a whole meal while driving to the next appointment? I've taken whole meals on planes, into business meetings, to school plays....

Consider your meal a big snack, and you'll get what you need to change your body.

You must eat, not snack. There is a big difference.

EAT

Are energy bars a good substitute for a meal?

AHHHHHHHHHHHHHHHHHH!

No, stop, look on the back of the wrapper on some of these energy bars.

Read the label and do the fat formula.

I picked one up the other day that was 29% fat. A candy bar—size serving of food with 29% fat!

You know what that is—that's what you call low-volume, high-fat crap, and that's exactly how we get fat.

A meal is a meal. An energy bar can be just about whatever they claim it to be.

I'll tell you the best energy bar you can get your hands on—

Thirty minutes of oxygen, and high-quality fuel.

Forget the energy bar—go get some food and oxygen into your body.

EAT

Some days I seem to be hungrier than other days. Why is this?

Let me jump right into the explanation of energy expended equals calories consumed.

Some days you do more than others.

Some days your body uses more fuel.

Some days you are more premenstrual than others.

And as your body gets fitter—if there is such a word—and stronger, it's developing in ways it never did in your unfit, no-energy days.

Three more reasons:

1. Your body uses fuel to increase muscle size.
2. An efficient metabolism processes fuel differently than a metabolic rate that functions like a slug.
3. And—a fit body gets hungry.

FEED IT!

Eating when you are hungry, drinking when you are thirsty—very sane. The more you do, the hungrier you'll be—very sane.

EAT

Should I eat when I'm not hungry?

No, never, ever.
Eat when you are hungry.
Drink when you are thirsty.
When you are not hungry, why would you eat?

EAT

Why do you say I should eat breakfast, even if it's not right when I get up?

Break the fast with high-quality fuel so that your body has energy to go on. It's a good idea when you think about it.

What a difference in my outlook on everything as well as my energy to bound out of bed and get my workday started.
— K.J., Nevada

EAT

Do I need to drink eight glasses of water a day?

I want to meet the bozo who made this diet tidbit up.

How about we clear this up once and for all? If drinking eight glasses of water a day had anything to do with burning body fat and increasing lean muscle mass, then count me in, I'm buoyant, water is my life, call me Esther Williams II.

It doesn't.

Sure, when you're thirsty, drink—and try and get a little water in once in a while. It's better for you than soda. But come on. . . .

Force-feeding eight glasses of water a day makes you go to the bathroom a lot, puts a strain on your bladder, and has nothing to do with reducing body fat. Let me ask you guys a question: Has it worked so far?

EAT

Are diet sodas okay to drink?

Sure, once in a while, if you don't mind the chemicals, colorings, and all the other stuff they're made of. But if you're drinking ten, fifteen, twenty of them a day—that's a problem. I've spoken with some diet soda drinkers who can't do without them—well, as with anything, if you can't live without it, you've got a problem.

We are the only nation on earth that not only volunteers for starvation, but pays millions of dollars for it every year.

EAT

Is it okay to drink coffee or things with caffeine in them?

Well, I sure as heck hope so because I do.

I think it's fair to say that caffeine, sugar, sodium, and rock 'n' roll—no, only kidding—fit in the category of "Nothing wrong with it as long as you don't live on it," or have a condition that caffeine aggravates.

Coffee is coffee.

Caffeine is not great.

There are some considerations—water-filtered is better than chemical-filtered, organic is better than processed junk, and as with anything, there is quality and there is crap. But that's not really the problem.

The real issue is answering this question is to ask a question: How much are you drinking? Is it one cup a day or 30? Easy to answer that—one cup of coffee a day is okay; 30 cups a day is way, way too much.

EAT

What about alcohol? Is it okay to have a drink?

Alcohol. It's a big subject to tackle in such a small book. There is no fat in alcohol. Alcohol got a bad rap in the diet industry because it's highly caloric for a small amount of no-nutritional-value stuff. And, in the old, old days of calorie counting, that glass of wine used up a lot of your daily calories.

But let's talk here. Alcohol is the most abused, socially acceptable drug in this country. It is responsible for thousands of deaths each year, and it is not conducive to a healthy lifestyle. I think all of us know what it feels like the morning after too much to drink—it's not as if you wake up and say, "Hey, I think I'll go get some exercise now."

So be careful. If you've got a problem, get some help. Don't worry or be embarrassed—millions of people are chemically dependent. You are not alone.

If you're asking about having a glass of wine or a beer with your chips and hot sauce at your favorite Mexican restaurant, and you're concerned about the fat content, keep your beer or wine and hot sauce, bag the chips, replace them with some corn or flour tortillas to dip into the sauce, and have a great time.

(But don't drive drunk—because if you hit my child, I'm gonna come after you . . . !)

EAT

Are fish and chicken okay to eat? Is one better than the other?

Well, that really depends who you listen to. I just read a book that explains what happens in the chicken factories—and right now I'd have to say NO, they're gross. But put that information aside for a moment, and let's get on with the issue: FAT.

Chicken may be lower in fat than red meat, and some fish is low in fat (but not all—do the fat formula on salmon and some other fish, and you'll be amazed).

Your lifestyle and personal preference are very much a part of the answer to this question. The more I read, the more experts I talk with, the further away from eating chicken I get. However, that's my deal, not yours. If it's chicken you want and it's fat you're concerned with, chicken is lower in fat than red meat.

EAT

Is all chicken the same? White meat, dark meat?

Not all chickens are created equal.
Dark meat is higher in fat than white.
With skin or skinless makes a difference.
Different cuts mean higher or lower quality.

If you're gonna eat it, you've got to do some investigating.

*Alone we can do so little; together we can do
so much.*
—Helen Keller

EAT

Can I eat red meat? I really love steak.

Sure you can, but you can't eat low-fat meat because there's no such thing. A lean steak is a contradiction in terms. Red meat is a high-fat food no matter how you cut it (pardon the pun!).

You can lower the fat a bit by trimming all you can, making sure the steak you're eating isn't loaded with "marbling"—you know, the fat "marbled" into the meat. There are high-fat cuts of meat and lower-fat cuts, and depending on what you choose, you can go from really, really high-fat to just high-fat. But the bottom line with red meat is that it's loaded with fat, and it's saturated fat—the fat that sticks to the inside of your arteries. (Yecch!)

Like ice cream, red meat is high-fat, no matter how you look at it.

Your body isn't manufacturing fat; it's coming from the end of your fork.

EAT

Won't I always be hungry without eating meat? How do I get full?

Full?

Ask someone who's just polished off a veggie burger loaded with lettuce, tomatoes, onions, pickles, a huge plate of fries (baked, not fried) slathered in rich tomato sauce, a cold pasta salad with cucumbers and peppers, three glasses of fresh lemonade, and marble cocoa cake for dessert.

Go ahead—ask me, because that's what I just had for lunch.

If it's full you want, then it's full you're gonna be.

Meat's got nothing to do with full; food does—and there's plenty of good-tasting, filling, high-volume, low-fat real food out there to fill your belly.

EAT

What does high fiber mean?

With fiber.

Not stripped of all nutrients and value.

Something that has come from the vine, the tree, or the earth to you—without being destroyed.

An apple vs. white sugar.

Brown rice vs. rice in seconds.

Fresh and raw vs. canned, frozen, or cooked to death.

You know—real food vs. fake.

EAT

I hate rice and beans—what else can I eat?

What's the deal with rice and beans? When in anything I've ever done did I say that rice and beans was the only thing you could eat????????

I'd hate rice and beans too if I thought it was all I could eat. BLAH......

"Anything" is the answer to this question. "What do you like?" would be my question to you.

What do I mean by "anything"?

Cereal	Bagels
Soups	Salads
Casseroles	Stews
Sandwiches	Hoagies
Pasta	Potatoes

and much, much more!

This time I know it's different. I love the food I eat. I don't feel deprived and this is how I want to live!
—C.R., Mississippi

EAT

I love pizza and Mexican food. Will I have to give these up forever?

I love, love, love Mexican food—and pizza, don't ask! My kids and I had the biggest pizza you've ever seen the other night with grilled veggies aplenty on top.

Pizza is fine without that one special ingredient that is loaded with saturated fat—cheese. Mexican food is fabulous—have your bean burritos, but check it out. If your beans are cooked in lard, like they are in many Mexican restaurants, they are loaded with fat.

Ask your waiter—and if their beans are cooked in lard, ask them to prepare you some without the fat. They'll understand, believe me, when they know that you know that they use bacon grease, lard, chicken fat, or whatever else to cook their beans—and they won't want you announcing it to everyone.

Those poor vegans—you know, that means vegetarians—or heart patients who think they are eating low-fat when they give up beef for beans—if only they knew what they are eating is just as bad. . . .

If they'd ask, they'd know.

Learning how to eat is not about dependence; it's about independence.

EAT

Will high-fiber food give me gas?

Probably, if it's been years since you've eaten anything other than nutritionally stripped, processed sugary junk. . . .

Then, yeah, put a little fiber in your diet and your body may react a bit until it gets used to real food.

Will high-fiber food give you gas for life and keep you indoors because your gas can't be trusted in public?

ABSOLUTELY NOT. It's a whole lot easier for your body to get used to real food than you think. It's gonna be thrilled to have something to live on.

EAT

What about bread?

What about bread, wonderful, filling, tasty bread?

Just as with anything that's made up of different ingredients, you've got to read your label and see what's in it.

Is your bread made from organic whole wheat flour, water, salt, yeast—or is your bread made with butter, bleached white flour, milk, sugar, salt, with some yeast thrown in?

You decide which is higher in quality and lower in fat. It's not difficult—just read, make the best choice for you and your family, and EAT BREAD.

EAT

Do I need to limit the amount of bread I eat?

You need to limit the amount of processed food you eat, and bread is a processed food. It doesn't grow that way—ever seen a bread tree?

Eat a sandwich, have two or three if you're particularly hungry, but living on bread is not a good idea.

The more whole foods (as close to the original food as possible), you get, the more value you're gonna get, and the better the fuel.

The better the fuel, the better the performance.

The better the performance, the faster and easier the results, and that's my goal—to get you the results you want.

There's nothing I like more than a couple of pieces of toast and jelly, or cinnamon bread, or french toast made without the egg yolks, but don't eat the whole loaf instead of eating other foods.

There are so many other foods you need to eat to get your body what it needs to keep going, so don't fill up on bread alone.

There's too much great food out there—save the room!

EAT

What about waffles and pancakes?

They are great!

Stacks of blueberry pancakes, whole wheat pancakes, hot and steamy and dripping in syrup. . . .

It's a close second to buckets of popcorn and an old movie on a rainy afternoon.

Isn't food wonderful when you don't have to be afraid of it?

But remember: Not all foods are created equal.

You've got to look at the ingredients, read the label, and know what you're eating. There are high-fat pancakes and low-fat pancakes!

EAT

Where can I get ideas about what to eat?

The minute you understand the concept of high-volume, low-fat, high-quality eating, you'll find yourself being drawn to every cookbook, magazine article, food guide, and new recipe that you could imagine.

You'll see a potato recipe and you'll go nuts! Pasta, veggies, rice, soups, casseroles, sandwich fixings—all of them will make you crazy. You'll probably have to modify some of the recipes you *do* find until the world catches up with your brilliance, but that's easy.

Use your imagination, and *Mangia*—that's Italian for EAT!—I think.

I hear and I forget. I see and I remember. I do and I understand.
　　　　　　　　　　　　　　　　　　　—Chinese proverb

EAT

Do I have to be a vegetarian?

I say respectfully to all the nonmeat eaters out there—some of the most unhealthy, fat, unbelievably unfit people I've ever met have been vegans.

Please spare me! If you don't want to cut up the cow, it's your business.

But fat makes you fat, whether it's the fat of the slaughtered animal or that of the hand-picked-in-love organic avocado.

EAT

Am I going to have to start shopping at health food stores to find things to eat?

God, no!

Health food people don't have the answer, and a lot of them have gross hair and never wear makeup. (I mean, how could you go through life never, ever putting on makeup? It's foreign to me!)

No. No. No. High-volume, low-fat food is available everywhere.

Living in a perfect bubble of health and fitness is not for me.

EAT

What is organic, and is it lower-fat?

Organic means grown or raised without chemicals.

Organic means not fed antibiotics or hormones.

Organic means higher quality, but it doesn't always mean low-fat.

That organically raised slab of beef is high-fat, with or without the chemicals.

EAT

Do I have to eat my rice and beans at the same time to get a complete protein?

You've been reading those food-combining books of the past or listening to your doctor (who took six weeks of nutrition in medical school), haven't you?

No.

FOOD-COMBINING UPDATE: In order to get a complete protein from a non-meat source, all you have to do is at any time of the day eat some kind of grain and bean, and you're set.

EAT

Here are some combinations I love:

Bean Burritos
Black Beans and Rice
Red Bean Chili with Rice
Boston Baked Beans on Toast
Lentils and Brown Rice Soup
Bean Taco
Split Pea Soup with Brown Rice
Bean and Grain Casserole

These are just a few bean and grain examples. There are lots more.

EAT

My husband only likes to eat meat and potatoes. How can I eat this way and still cook for him?

A couple of options here:

Eat the potatoes, not the steak?

Explain to your husband that if he keeps doing the meat, potatoes, and gravy he-man kind of meal, he may not be around very long?

Show him a video of someone having a heart attack? Perhaps the pain and intensity of the whole thing may convince him to start eating the potatoes and including something a little lower in fat than the steak?

Make your own decisions about your own life, health, lifestyle, body, and wellness, because it's *your* life we are talking about, and *your* life is precious.

Maybe he'll follow your lead . . .

EAT

I've heard you say to check ingredients on the package label. I know to look for butter and oil, but is there something else I should be looking for?

SUGAR.

The big ingredient in low-fat and nonfat foods. Those sneaky buggers—my pet name for the food manufacturers—don't have the courage just to say LOADED WITH SUGAR. You'll find as you are reading your labels that sugar can be listed in 10 different ways on one label.

Sucrose. Fructose. Malt sweetener. Honey. Dextrols. All different names for the same thing—sugar.

You also might want to check the quality of the food you are buying, as you develop more consumer awareness savvy. You may want to start checking for preservatives, colorings, chemicals—but that's your deal, and may not be your concern.

What you are going to find is, the more you learn, the more informed you are, the more your choices, concerns, considerations, and needs will change.

It's a wonderful process.

EAT

Is honey better for me than sugar?

As much as the health food store folks want you to believe it is, it isn't.

Honey is sugar.

Sugar is sugar, and we eat way too much of it.

Everyone says I look great. They ask me what diet I'm on. I tell them I'm not on a diet.
—F.R., Connecticut

EAT

How about a little cream in my coffee? Is that so bad?

So bad? There is no bad or good—there's only high-fat or low-fat.

That little bit of cream is high-fat.

It's not as if you can never have cream again—you choose your battles—but if you have the cream in your coffee *with* the cinnamon roll for breakfast, the burger and fries for lunch, and the steak with creamy dressing for dinner, you are looking at trouble.

Cream is high-fat, but there are plenty of low-fat white creamy alternatives for coffee. Think about what you are willing or not willing to give up—and make your own decision.

How about having a little cream in your coffee, along with oatmeal, whole wheat toast, and a fruit plate for breakfast? Now we are talking high-volume.

It's not all or nothing anymore—that's diet stuff.

It's high-fat vs. low-fat.

High-fat makes you fat; low-fat helps keep you lean and healthy.

EAT

What can I use when baking instead of butter or margarine?

Water.

Applesauce.

Check out the million and one cookbooks on the market that give you a million and one substitutes for baking low-fat.

You can make a high-fat blueberry muffin or a low-fat blueberry muffin—it's all in the ingredients (pardon the pun). Enjoy—and send me a tin of them. I love muffins.

EAT

Isn't margarine better for me than butter?

You'd think it was, wouldn't you, based on advertising? How those margarine manufacturers got this into our brains is something we should all study—a course in brainwashing!!!

Do the fat formula—but watch out, it's gonna make you crazy when you see how high in fat margarine is.

Never doubt that a small group of thoughtful, committed citizens can change the world. Indeed, it is the only thing that ever has.

—Margaret Mead

EAT

Is it okay to eat butter sometimes?

Sometimes is no different from all the time, as far as percentage of fat is concerned. If you are eating a tub of butter or a teaspoon of butter, it's still 100% fat.

But—living on butter and having it once a week are two totally different things.

It's your choice.

EAT

Isn't it okay to use olive oil?

That virgin stuff. The fuel of the Greek goddess!

Okay, or better to use? Well, no better than any other food that's 100% fat. Yep, all oil is 100% fat, no matter how you look at it.

Some oils are higher quality than others. Some are more expensive. Some are saturated fat, some unsaturated. But all oil is 100% fat.

If you are making that fabulous pasta salad, loaded with fresh veggies, spices, herbs, buckets of it, ready to eat, you don't have to worry about fat—unless, of course, you add virgin olive oil or any other kind of oil. Then you've got one ingredient that's 100% fat in your very low-fat, high-volume, high-quality meal.

Why do it when there are so many alternatives to oil? Olive or not olive, if it's 100% fat, that speaks for itself.

EAT

Isn't pasta sauce—marinara sauce—low-fat?

Wow—hold on. Don't assume that for a second.
Tomatoes are low-fat, the herbs and spices that
season the stuff are low-fat, but the oil that's in some
of these sauces isn't anywhere near low-fat.

If you're at a restaurant, ask them how much oil,
chicken stock, lard, bacon grease, or whatever else
they may put into some of these sauces that go on
top of a perfectly low-fat plate of pasta.

If it's store-bought—read, read, read the label.
Don't assume because it's a tomato sauce that it's
low-fat. As a matter of fact, don't assume anything.

Read, learn, and make your own choices—

What you'll find is that there are some great low-
fat sauces out there.

EAT

How can I make my food taste good? Without butter it seems so bland.

Taste good?????!!!! Salt, pepper, garlic, soy sauce, hot sauce, herbs, sauces, dressings out the ying-yang (that's not the name of some metaphysical sauce, I mean literally out the wazoo!). Even butter has its substitutes, although some of them are a little scary.

There are so many ways to make high-volume, low-fat food taste good that don't make you fat or contribute to heart disease like butter does. . . .

You never know—your imagination might start running wild and you may come up with your own low-fat taste-adder, and then you can contact me and we can mass-market it and you'll have your face on a sauce like Paul Newman and then . . . . the world!

Experiment. . . .

Use your imagination.

I make choices every day that make an enormous difference in my life.

EAT

Aren't baked potatoes fattening?
They're starch.

That's not even diet thinking; that's 1950s thinking.

Before our leaders in nutrition knew any better, they taught us that starch was fattening, which made us all very afraid of the bread, potatoes, pastas. . . . All of it was the worst thing we could put into our bodies if we were worried about getting fat.

So we didn't eat the bread, we cut way back on calories, we drank our milk, and we spread our butter all over everything but starch. . . .

No—baked potatoes are *not* fattening.

A baked potato stuffed with the thousands of low-fat things you can stuff it with is an easy, high-volume, low-fat quality food.

ENJOY!

EAT

How can I keep things from sticking to the pan without using oil?

- Use a nonstick pan.
- Saute in water.
- Use vegetable broth. (Check the label, though—
  not all veggie broths are created equal, and
  many have too much fat.)
- Bake.
- Stew.
- Broil.

Whatever....

EAT

Can I drink fruit juice?

Sure, if you like it. Can you live on it? Is that your breakfast, a glass of juice? No, no, no.

Have your food, and have a glass of juice if you'd like. But check out the amount of sugar in some of these commercial juices, and if you want to try something different, try juicing your own. You'll be amazed at what you can make—fruits, vegetables, all kinds of things turn into juice.

If you like it, drink it, but remember: you gotta eat, eat, eat, eat.

You can begin to "Stop the Insanity" in your life by eating.

EAT

What about fruit? How much of it should I eat?

There is no "should" when it comes to eating fruit. Fruit is a food, like many other foods. Some people like it more than others. Fruit has been touted in the days of dieting as the thing to eat, especially for breakfast. I'm not sure why, since fruit is fast-burning (it's sugar)—that's not gonna give you all the energy you need to get through your morning, but those were the diet days and those boys got a lot of things wrong.

Fruit is good. If you enjoy it, eat it. If it's been 20 years since you included an apple in your day, you might want to consider including it more often. But if it's breakfast you're eating, have your cereal, toast, some fruit, a glass of juice, tea, or coffee or whatever you like—

Now, that's a BREAKFAST!

EAT

I'm pregnant. Can I still eat this way?

AHHHHHHHHHHHHHH. Never, ever, ever, ever is it more important that you get oxygen every day, have a healthy percent of lean muscle mass and body fat, and be strong and healthy than when you are responsible for the health of another human being . . . your baby.

Should you eat high-quality foods while you are pregnant? Absolutely. This way of eating is a healthy, good way, not a special program or diet. Ask your doctor—and if he/she doesn't get it, find a new doctor.

CONGRATULATIONS . . . and be healthy.

*Shared joy is double joy, and shared sorrow
is half-sorrow.*
                                        —Swedish proverb

EAT

***I'm diabetic. Is it okay for me to follow a
low-fat, high-volume, high-quality diet like
you suggest?***

It's a whole lot more than okay.

It's the most important thing you can do for yourself. Hasn't your doctor told you how important the
connection between what you're eating and being a
diabetic is? Surely he or she has suggested you
change the way you are eating—increasing the quality of your foods, cutting back on the foods that are
directly connected to your disease, decreasing your
body fat, and increasing your strength and health so
that your body is strong and able to deal with your
disease.

And surely you've received suggestions and reading material about your options, so that you can
make intelligent decisions about something that affects your life. I hope he's mentioned Dr. John
McDougall, and the wonderful work that he does
with health and nutrition.

There's so much terrific information out there, and
so many ways to support your body so that you can
live a high-quality life with your diabetes. Who
knows what could happen when you give your body
what it needs, and start solving some of the problems instead of living with the symptoms.

EAT

I love popcorn. Is it healthy?

Popcorn—buckets of it—and an old tear-jerker movie on a rainy afternoon—what could be better?

I love popcorn too, but you've got to put on your fat detective hat in a big way when it comes to some of the packaged popcorn on the market today.

Do the fat formula on some of them—especially some of the leading "diet" brands of popcorn. It will blow your mind. Some of them are as high as 57% fat. . . .

Popcorn, 57% fat? It's impossible—unless the manufacturer makes it 57% fat, because popcorn is a low-fat, fabulous-tasting, crunchy, perfect movie-watching snack.

Oh, and the next time you're at the movie theater, ask the snack bar manager to show you the packet of yellow fat that they make the popcorn with . . . .

YUKKKKKKKKKK.

EAT

You always talk about keeping a "feedbag" of snacks in your car. What do you keep in it?

Me and my feedbag—could be a movie-of-the-week or maybe a country-western song. I carry food everywhere I go. In my car, on airplanes, in hotels, at the movies—wherever I am, you can bet there's food. I keep all kinds of travel foods in my feedbag; bagels, pretzels, low-fat potato chips, pasta salads (no oil, of course), crackers, dried fruit, trail mix (low-fat, of course)—anything that is low-fat and anything that is crunchy and salty because I love crunchy and salty.

If you want to be healthy, you must eat.

EAT

I'm afraid to go out and eat because I don't know what to eat.

Afraid no more—that's what we'll call you from now on.

All you have to do is scan the menu for all the high-volume, low-fat foods you see.

Then you've got to ask the waiter for capers, spices, hot sauces, Worcestershire sauce, Cajun anything, because that's a great taste, or whatever taste you are in the mood for—and make your own concoctions.

Mush it up, spice it up, throw it all together, and you've got a high-volume, low-fat meal, while everyone else in the restaurant is eating more fat in one meal than we should put into our bodies in a month.

You'll be getting leaner and they'll be getting fatter, even though everybody's eating in the same place.

EAT

How do I know what I order in a restaurant is low-fat?

You don't, and never will—unless you ask.

Ask the waiter what is in the marinara sauce.

Get the ingredients in the salad dressing.

And here's the big one, the question that forces wonderful, honest waiters and waitresses into a life of lying: "Is there any oil in this dish?"

Oh, they'll tell you no, believing there isn't, and then when the dish comes you'll see those little oil bubbles floating on top of your soup, your main dish will be floating side to side on the dish on a greasy surface of oil, and no matter how much they insist the chef didn't put any oil into your food, all you gotta do is touch it—that's it, stick your fingers in that food and rub them together—that greasy, high-fat, shiny stuff, that's oil, and as many times as you have to send it back, send it back—

UNTIL YOU GET WHAT YOU WANT.

It's your money, it's your health, and it's your daily fat intake.

So—

ASK.

EAT

Is there a difference between Italian and Chinese food?

Ask an Italian, and he'll tell you there is.

Ask me, and I'll tell you that as far as high-volume, low-fat eating is concerned, both are equal.

PASTA—a bonus in any restaurant. Use a little imagination, some fresh herbs, tomatoes, onions, capers, veggies, and mix it all together for the best pasta dish you've ever had—without the fat.

CHINESE—who doesn't love Chinese food? It's the best—and it's also some of the highest-fat food around, unless you lie. Yep, lie big. I tell every waiter/waitress that I order from, especially in Chinese restaurants, that I'm allergic to all oils.

I've come close to having a fake seizure when they bring me a dish, insisting there is no oil—and my fingers sliding together are telling me there are tons of oil all over my food.

You've got to ask.

You've got to get what you want.

Most important, you've got to know that there isn't a restaurant you *can't* eat in, because you can always throw together a high-volume, low-fat meal, even if it looks a little odd, and your waiter/waitress thinks you're a loon. . . .

Who cares, you'll be a lean loon.

EAT

Are any of the fast-food restaurants good?

I eat at them all the time when I'm on the road. I've been to towns in the last couple of years where the local fast-food restaurant is the only place to go out and get a bite to eat.

There's always that famous baked potato and all the stuffings from the salad bar. The high-volume, low-fat selection in some of these places is not much, but I've always been able to find something to eat.

A man has to be Joe McCarthy to be called ruthless. All a woman has to do is put you on hold.
> —Marlo Thomas

EAT

How many calories can I eat?

More than you ever could have dreamed. Here's the chart, but remember, it's only an indication of the amount of fuel you need, based on your energy expended, to maintain body fat percentage, good health, and to have enough energy to get through the day.

EAT

Daily Caloric Consumption Predictions for Women*

Pounds	Resting Calories "Doing Nothing"	Low Activity Low-Impact Walking or Cycling 2–3 Times a Week	Medium Activity Low-Impact Walking or Cycling 4–5 Times a Week	High Activity Low-Impact Walking or Cycling 6–7 Times a Week	
100	1,120	1,450	1,570	1,680	
110	1,150	1,490	1,600	1,720	
120	1,190	1,550	1,670	1,780	
130	1,220	1,580	1,700	1,830	
140	1,250	1,630	1,750	1,880	
150	1,280	1,660	1,800	1,920	
160	1,320	1,720	1,850	1,980	
170	1,350	1,750	1,890	2,000	
180	1,380	1,790	1,930	2,070	
190	1,420	1,850	1,990	2,100	
200	1,450	1,880	2,030	2,180	
210	1,480	1,950	2,050	2,200	
220	1,513	1,970	2,100	2,270	
230	1,540	2,000	2,160	2,300	
240	1,580	2,050	2,200	2,400	
250	1,610	2,090	2,250	2,410	
260	1,640	2,130	2,300	2,460	
270	1,676	2,170	2,350	2,500	
280	1,710	2,220	2,400	2,560	
290	1,740	2,260	2,440	2,600	
300	1,770	2,480	2,500	2,660	

*Individuals running or exercising at high intensities may need more calories.
Modified and adapted from Oliver Owen, "Resting metabolic requirements of men and women," *Mayo Clinic Report*, volume 163 (1988), and "A reappraisal of caloric requirements in healthy women," *American Journal of Clinical Nutrition*, volume 44 (1986): 1–19.

EAT

I weigh over 400 pounds—off the charts for calorie consumption. How do I know how much to eat?

All you have to do is burn the fat. So what if it's 400 pounds worth of fat—burning fat is burning fat, and we all gotta do the same thing.

The daily calorie consumption chart is an indicator of how much people need to eat based on their activity level. These are not figures etched in gold. If you are taking in a couple thousand calories a day, you'll be fine, as long as the calories you are taking in are low-fat and—Okay, I won't say it again because you guys know what else the food needs to be. . . .

Take in the fuel, begin to move within your level of fitness (which at 400 pounds is nearly nonexistent—that's okay, because at 260 pounds, mine was too), and you'll start to burn the fat, increase your strength, get your body functioning at a different level, and feel and look better than you could ever imagine.

Eat when you're hungry. Regular meals. Great food. Low, low fat. And get some oxygen and some strengthening and bingo—you've got it down. The fat, that is.

Be well, and enjoy!

EAT

Do I need to watch the amount of sodium I eat?

I know I do three days before my period because all I think about and want to eat is salt.

By the end of the second day of those wonderful couple of anxiety-for-no-reason days, I'm the Goodyear blimp because of the amount of sodium I've consumed, and that's not good.

Sure, we all need to watch the amount of sodium we eat. Just as with sugar, we eat too much of it. Many people need to watch sodium for more important reasons than not wanting to look like the Goodyear blimp—medical considerations, for one.

There are plenty of wonderful, low-fat, tasty spices, herbs, and sprinkle-on-your-food items crammed on the grocery shelf to use as a salt replacement or to cut back a bit.

Give them a try. See what you think.

EAT

What can I do when I really crave sweets and chocolate?

Eat sweets. Blow the chocolate off. Chocolate is high-fat, and that low-fat chocolate stuff that's out there is the grossest-tasting stuff around.

But there are plenty of sweet, low-fat items available. Again, go for quality, not chemical concoctions loaded with 20 different kinds of sugar. The only way to know, of course, is to be the fat-detective, label-reading, intelligent consumer that you are, and make the best choice.

If you want something sweet, eat something sweet, but don't exclude the meal for the ringy-dingy-dongy snack—that's not food, and won't keep you going all day.

Making better choices will help change your body.

EAT

I like candy. Can I eat it?

Someone said to me recently that they'd been eating bags and bags of their favorite little candies because they were low in fat.

Guys—no matter how you cut it, you can't eat bags and bags of candy.

It's not real food.

That's a hell of a lot of useless calories that should be coming from real fuel.

Sugar by the ton isn't good, and bags of skootles—come on. . . .

Yes, you can eat candy if it's low-fat, and you want it once in a while, after your huge high-volume, low-fat meal.

Or you can have it as a snack, once in a while, when you're premenstrual.

But bags and bags of it—that's the problem.

EAT

What about nuts? Are they good for me?

They are very high in fat, and high-fat is NOT good for you.

My most rewarding private moment was when I looked in the mirror and I had only one chin—it made me smile.

—B.P., Utah

EAT

When I go to parties, I can't seem to stay away from the food table. What can I do?

Don't go to the party.

Or, go so full that you can't think of eating?

Or, understand that you *can* stay away from the food table. It's your decision, the table is not pulling you in with some invisible force field, and you have the ability to not eat.

Hey—there's something happening that's gonna make your party-going food experience a lot easier. People are becoming more conscious and serving high-volume, low-fat food at their parties. Start the trend with your circle of friends and you won't have the problem—

Then, you can eat!

EAT

I don't have a lot of money and can't afford to buy expensive special foods. What can I eat?

That's wonderful. Not that you don't have a lot of money—that's hard—but it's wonderful that you can't buy special expensive foods, because you don't have to.

The high-volume, low-fat foods that I'm talking about are cheaper than buying the steak and specialty foods. A lot of them come in bulk so you can get them dirt cheap. Check out your local health food store's bulk bins—you wouldn't believe what you can do with a couple of dollars and a bucket full of pasta, rice, barley, millet. . . . All right, maybe you're not ready for millet, but it's cheap, high-volume, low-fat, and versatile!

You will never need specialty, prepackaged, diet, gross, frozen expensive foods again.

Now we have to help you make a living. . . .

We're working on it (pardon the pun)—more opportunity for women. Give me some time and we'll talk.

EAT

Can my whole family eat this way? Do children need more fat than adults?

Childhood obesity is a national epidemic in this country. Children after the age of two don't need any more fat than adults, and they, like the adults in our country, are getting way, way, way too much.

Obesity isn't the only issue when you are talking about fat and kids.

Heart disease is another very important factor. Heart disease doesn't start when you're fifty-five; it starts when you're two, three, four years old.

You know what else is directly connected to heart disease? Saturated FAT, cholesterol, lack of activity—lifestyle, lifestyle, lifestyle.

Please, let's stop feeding the children high-fat, processed, nutritionally depleted crap, and let's get them some high-volume, low-fat food and go for a walk together. The advantages of being well and physically fit apply to children just like adults.

We owe them that.

Whatever you do to your child's body, you do to your child's mind.
—Penelope Leach

EAT

I'm making an effort to cut back on my daily fat intake by drinking 2% instead of whole milk, but I'm not getting leaner. Why?

Now, watch me get a little passionate/mad here.

It's people like you who are making the effort and being deceived that really gets my goat. (What in the world does that expression mean . . . ???)

I hate to be the one to break it to you, but that 2% milk you are drinking is not 2%—it's 32%, which is not and never will be low-fat.

I know—your trusted brand! They said 2% and you believed them.

Your heart, your arteries, your thighs. . . .

Yep, you've been lied to. I'm sorry, but better than sorry is the fat detective way out. Use the fat formula, and uncover the truth.

Don't ever, ever believe a label. Do the formula and see for yourself.

Then, and only then, will you know that you are taking in low-fat.

Then, and only then, will you start to get leaner.

Unfortunately, sometimes people don't hear you until you scream.

—Stefanie Powers

EAT

How do I get the kids to change their diets?

Not by walking in one day and announcing that they will never eat fat again.

Slowly, respectfully.

When you put the chicken dinner in front of them, throw in a grain dish. They won't scream, "UGH, IT'S A GRAIN!!" They'll eat both.

Instead of spaghetti and meatballs, try spaghetti and turkey balls.

You can cut back on your family's fat intake and nobody will know the difference—until they all start looking and feeling better.

EAT

What do I pack in my children's lunches?

Anything they like. Chips, sandwiches, salads, fruit—I don't know, what do they enjoy? Kids are no different than you and I. They like what tastes good. Their tastes are as individual as they are, and they need high-quality fuel, movement, and oxygen just as much—if not more, because they are developing at such a fast pace—as we do.

Whatever they like.

EAT

I hate to cook. Are diet frozen dinners okay to eat?

You decide. Read the label. If putting 97 things that you can't pronounce into your body doesn't bother you, then it's okay.

Check your fat content. Do the fat formula on your frozen diet dinner and see if the fat percentage is the percentage you want in your daily intake.

Check out the quantity of food. If that's all you want to eat, then it's okay.

But you don't have to love to cook to eat well. Throwing a potato in a pot is not cooking; it's throwing a potato in a pot.

The way you eat is your decision. The consequences of the way you eat are your consequences. It's up to you whether it's okay or not.

I think I have tried every diet food, packaged meal, and pills at least once. I wouldn't dare say how much I spent on them. But as far as the food goes, the picture on the box would probably taste better.
—P.T., Texas

EAT

I am a busy working mom who doesn't have much time to cook. Do you have any suggestions for quick meals?

It's all quick these days, because who has time for anything else? One nifty trick I've found is to cook one day a week. Make a couple of soups, casseroles, sauces, pack them up in plastic containers, and let them sit in the fridge all week.

When you rush home every night, it only takes a second to make pasta, rice, or whatever it is you want to add to, place under, or fill up with.

The other night I had a leftover rice dish with veggies and soy sauce mixed in, and I put it into the whole wheat tortillas, topped it all off with hot sauce, put a few low-fat chips on the plate with a couple of ears of corn, and my kids thought I was a genius. One of my sons said, "Hey, Mom, this tastes like we went out to dinner at the best Mexican restaurant in town!"

I took all the credit for the meal from start to finish—about 20 minutes in the making (the damn corn took the longest to cook!).

EAT

I only have 10 to 15 pounds to lose. Is this a good way for me to eat?

Why wouldn't it be? Your 10 to 15 pounds is no different than someone else's 100. It's all the same, and there's only one way on earth to change it. You gotta eat, you gotta breathe, and you gotta move if you want to get lean, strong, and healthy.

Same process, less fat to burn.

This is not a diet. This is about balancing your daily caloric intake with your energy expended, and getting well.

EAT

I'm an emotional eater and I'm afraid that this won't work for me because I'll still binge.

Everyone is an emotional eater. There isn't a person on earth who doesn't connect food to emotion. If you have an eating disorder, you need to get help—and there's tons of help available now that our society has come out of the eating disorder closet.

While you are getting help with your eating disorder, what's the matter with eating higher-quality food? I mean, respectfully, if you're going to binge, why not binge on better-quality fuel?

I have an opinion about recovery. Anyone who is recovering from anything—depression, chemical dependency, eating disorders—should be getting oxygen, building strength, and improving the quality of their fuel even more than the rest of us. When you're trying to recover, you deserve and need all the help you can get—and this helps.

EÄT

If my arteries are clogged with fat from eating all this high-fat food, will they ever get better if I start eating low-fat?

Oh, how wonderful—you are going to get healed.

You're going to love and respect your body so much when you see how brilliantly it comes back from the dead. Yes, you can clean up an artery. Sure, you can unclog what's clogged—the information is out and the experts now know that what you are eating is directly connected to the number one killer in this country: heart disease.

If you want to get the best info out there on heart disease, read Dr. Dean Ornish's book called *Reversing Heart Disease*. Check out the first word in the title: *reversing*.

Reverse, unclog, and LIVE.

I'm thrilled for you.

Let's stop the symptoms. Solve the problem!

EAT

Is there any food that burns fat fastest?

Food doesn't burn fat, other than contributing to the efficiency of your metabolic rate.

Aerobic exercise burns fat.

If there was any one thing we could all eat that burned away the fat, then we'd have the answer in a pill, an herb, a food, an energy bar. . . .

It ain't gonna happen, because there is only one way to change the way you look and feel—

You gotta eat, you gotta breathe, and you gotta move.

No food, no nothing, does what those three things do for you when it comes to health, wellness, and fat-burning.

EAT

Sometimes I look at thin people eating in restaurants and wonder why they can eat so much when everything I eat goes right to my hips and thighs. It doesn't seem fair.

What are you eating, and what are they eating? Are you glaring at the thinnies through the fried chicken, while they are busy being thin between bites of high-volume low-fat food?

Not many people can eat high-fat and not be fat or unhealthy, so even if the skinny minny is eating the fried chicken and is not morbidly obese, you know she's hurting inside.

Only one in a thousand people can eat anything they want and not gain weight—bully for them. It doesn't mean they don't have high cholesterol and are on the verge of a heart attack. It doesn't mean they aren't dying for energy and feel weak, depressed, and physically awful.

I consider the fat people of the world more honest . . . at least we show the world what we are. Those skinny-on-the-outside-eat-everything-they-want kind of people are deceptive—don't you think?

Do the hardest thing on earth for you. Act for yourself. Face the truth.
                                        —Katherine Mansfield

EAT

Can you ever "cheat" and get away with it?

Cheat what? Yourself, your health? Cheating is a diet mentality, and when you stop the insanity in your life and realize how easy it is, you'll forget about that cheating diet mentality forever. Cheating means you are only allowed certain things.

Look, if you "cheat" yourself and start eating fat, you'll get fat. But if you desire a certain taste, texture, sweet, sour, salty thing—have it, just try and make it as low-fat as you can get. Then you don't have to "cheat" yourself or your body of anything.

Show me a woman who doesn't feel guilty and I'll show you a man.

—Erica Jong

BREATHE

Without oxygen you die.
—Susan Powter

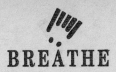

BREATHE

Talk about something we all take for granted.

OXYGEN.

Without it, you and I are goners. But we don't think about it, we don't spend any time on it, and we certainly don't get enough of it.

Oxygen is the most vital ingredient in wellness, and there is a way to get more of it into your life. That's what the BREATHE section is all about: we're gonna get you more energy, more oxygen into your body every day.

It's cheap, easy to get, and makes a whole lot of difference in your life.

Here's to energy!

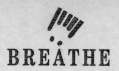

BREATHE

What's the deal with breathing 100 times a day? Is that really important?

Oxygen is the big cheese, Mr. Big—as we like to call oxygen and other things in my house (pet name for the husband, you know). Getting back into the habit of breathing is the most important beginning you can make if you want to get lean, strong, and healthy. Oxygen is the most vital ingredient in wellness.

For me, getting back into the habit of breathing meant thinking about it and doing it.

Just taking a breath in and blowing it out once in a while. Call me excessive—that meant doing it 100 times a day. Some days 80, some days 100, but I'll tell you, I thought about breathing and did it all day, and guess what happened? I got back into the habit of taking a breath.

Breathing. Don't ask. I do it all the time and it *does* help. It helps give you the energy you need to do what you've got to do. Remember, Oxygen equals Energy . . . so yeah, it's important in the beginning that you breathe 100 times a day.

Just to get back into the habit.

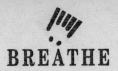

BREATHE

I thought I was breathing. What am I doing wrong?

Well, you are breathing—unless you're writing to me from beyond the grave.

But that doesn't mean you are getting enough oxygen into your body.

It doesn't mean that your body is fit enough to be distributing the oxygen properly.

And it doesn't mean that every cell and every muscle in your body is getting what it needs to live on.

So, breathe, move, build lean muscle mass and you'll be an oxygen distribution machine.

You'll feel the difference.

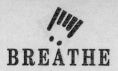

BREATHE

Is there a correct way to breathe?

Depends on who you talk to and what your goal is.

If you are trying to levitate, there probably is a special breathing technique, but—

If what you want is to get some oxygen into your body during exercise, then it really boils down to whatever works for you . . . as long as you breathe.

Some breathing experts suggest you breathe in through your nose and out through your mouth.

Some personal trainers suggest you exhale on the exertion and inhale on the release—and others suggest the exact opposite.

You know what I do?

I breathe. Anyway I want to.

Depending on how I'm feeling or what's going on at the time. If I have a stuffy nose, I breathe through my mouth the whole workout. If I'm feeling very focused and strong, I try different breathing patterns. If I am premenstrual, the best I can do is breathe when I think about it because I'm too confused to figure out much more than that.

Just think about it, and start breathing. . . .

Losing weight is a side effect of getting healthy.

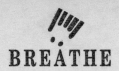

BREATHE

How do you know when you're "in oxygen"?

When you're not gasping for breath.

When you're not huffing and puffing. Not sucking wind.

When you're not blue in the face and wishing that your aerobic activity was over, hating every minute of it because you can't breathe, or feeling like you are about to die.

You can take your heart rate if you like, but the 60% to 80% target heart efficiency standard set by those black-and-red target heart rate charts in every aerobic classroom in the country only pertain to people who already have healthy resting heart rates. In other words, if you are not already fit, don't shoot for the target heart rate goal.

In oxygen means being able to carry on a conversation—not a lengthy chat, just able to respond if spoken to.

In oxygen means challenge your breathing but don't get out of breath. Being able to breathe is a good sign you're working within your fitness level.

In oxygen means you should be gaining strength and getting energy from the exercise because you're getting oxygen into your body.

In order to be aerobic and burn fat, you've got to be in oxygen. Not blue—but your natural color with a healthy glow.

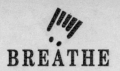

BREATHE

Why is it so important not to be out of oxygen?

Because you'll die if you're without oxygen for any length of time.

Because it's the fuel for every cell and muscle in your body.

Because it's the giver of life.

Because if you are out of oxygen while exercising, you are not aerobic, not fat-burning.

Because fat burns in oxygen.

So—if you want to burn the fat, you've got to be in. . . .

The big cheese.

Knowledge is not power. Getting the right information and learning to apply it to your life is power.

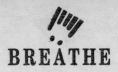

BREATHE

"Without oxygen, you die." What does that mean?

Well, it means just without oxygen, you die.

Think about what happens when your cells and muscles don't get enough oxygen.

There are a couple of ways to get oxygen into your body. One, carry around an oxygen tank and suck from it every few seconds. Cumbersome, but you'll get oxygen.

Or two: exercise, move.

There's the big bad death—that'll happen if you hold your breath for any length of time.

Then there's slow death—the kind that you live with every day when your body doesn't have enough oxygen.

Lack of energy.

Not thinking clearly.

Lethargic.

Depressed.

Unmotivated. . . .

On and on it goes until you get your body what it needs.

OXYGEN.

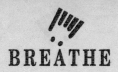

BREATHE

I heard you say "being in conversation" when you work out. Can you explain what this means?

Having a quick chat like, "Boy, is this fun!"
"Gee, I'm thirsty."
"Forty-five minutes up yet?"
"Keep moving."
Being able to answer a question if need be—
"Nope, fifteen minutes left."
"Damn, I forgot my water bottle!"
Not being out of breath.

It doesn't mean a constant stream of chatter or a lengthy conversation, just being able to respond.

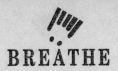

BREATHE

If you're supposed to be able to talk and exercise at the same time, how do you know when it's getting too easy and not burning fat?

Good question. Thirty minutes in oxygen doesn't mean having tea and chatting with a friend. In order to burn fat, you have to be aerobic, in oxygen, and have an elevated heart rate to get that blood pumping and the body burning fat. You know when it's easy and ineffective—that slow, shop-and-mall-walk that we've all done is not exercise.

Even if you definitely were in oxygen while writing the check for the outfit that cost more than you (or any of us) are willing to admit. . . .

You'll know when it's a breeze.—When it is, increase your level of intensity and build higher and higher . . .

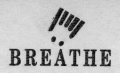

BREATHE

If I'm working out so hard that I'm gasping for air, doesn't it mean that I'm burning more fat because I'm working harder?

NOOOOOOOOOOOOOOOOOOOOOOOOOOOOOOOOOOOOOOOO!

It means you are gasping for air and not burning fat.

In order to burn fat, you must be in oxygen, not gasping for air.

Then, when you are cardiovascularly fit enough to go to the next level, you do—and you keep going until you're as fit as you want to be, or until you've burned off all the fat you want to burn off.

That's how you get fit and burn fat, not by beating the heck out of yourself.

Don't agonize, organize.
—Florynce Kennedy

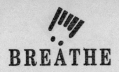

BREATHE

I smoked for 10 years and have recently quit. Will my breathing get better from working out?

Sure, your breathing is going to get better—*if* you work within your fitness level.

Don't get discouraged when you start to move and discover that within minutes you are finding it hard to breathe. Be realistic—you're starting out unfit, cardiovascularly weak, and you've just quit smoking.

Just decrease your level of intensity and stay in oxygen, and keep building the cardiovascular strength that your body so desperately needs, and getting your heart and lungs strong, clean, and healthy.

What a wonderful gift you've given yourself. Congratulations, be patient, listen to your body, and rebuild.

After about three weeks the weight sitting on my chest was gone. With a couple more weeks, it didn't hurt me to take a deep breath while I was walking. It's wonderful!!!

—A.J., Tennessee

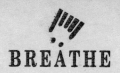

BREATHE

*I've been working out recently, and my
breathing seems to be getting better. Is
it my imagination?*

Imagination? Why would you say that?

Are you imagining more energy? More strength?

Your cells and muscles are screaming THANK
YOU FOR GIVING US THE FUEL WE LIVE
ON—WE FEEL SO MUCH BETTER AND WE CAN
DO MORE FOR YOU BECAUSE YOU ARE FEED-
ING US!

Your body is thrilled, getting healthier, feeling
better. . . .

You don't have an overactive imagination—you
have a healthier body.

Isn't it wonderful, and so easy!

*Men are taught to apologize for their weaknesses,
women for their strengths.*

—Lois Wyse

MOVE

I've been thin but never fit.
This time I'm going
to be fit.
—M.H., Oregon

MOVE

I know.

EXERCISE = TORTURE
EXERCISE = NEON
EXERCISE = LOUD MUSIC
EXERCISE = PAIN AND SUFFERING

Well, not anymore. Fitness is for everyone, any age, any weight. It's time to learn how to move within your fitness level so that you can burn some fat, increase your cardio-endurance and muscular strength, and get lean, strong, and healthy.

You can do it.

You'll change the way you look and feel, increase the quality of your life, and wake up every day with a foundation of wellness that will change your life.

MOVE

What is aerobic exercise?

The definition of aerobic is any movement in oxygen with an elevated heart rate for 30 minutes or more.

Walking.
Biking.
Hiking.
Swimming.
Rowing.
Whatever movement you enjoy....

Aerobic is fat-burning. Aerobic increases your metabolic rate, gets oxygen to every cell and muscle in your body, and does a whole lot more.
Aerobic IS NOT:

Loud music.
Fancy choreography.
Fancy leotards.
Big hair.

MOVE

What's the best aerobic exercise?

The one you enjoy doing.

If anyone had told me that jogging was the only way to get lean, strong, and healthy, I'd be 560 pounds now. I hated jogging then and I can't stand it now, so I wouldn't have done it. Doesn't do you a bit of good if you won't do it.

Find what you like, maybe a couple of things. Mix 'em up. Walk one day, bike the next, throw swimming in once a week—whatever you enjoy.

Do it for 30 minutes in oxygen with an elevated heart rate and you'll be burning that fat!!!!!!!!

MOVE

Why is aerobic exercise so important to losing fat?

Movement in oxygen with an elevated heart rate—otherwise known as aerobic activity—is fat-burning because fat burns in oxygen.

Fat is one of the fuels your body uses for energy.

The problem is, most of us have way, way too much fat stored and we're not burning it off. So it stores on our hips, thighs, butts, and stomachs, and the only way to get rid of it is to burn it off by doing an aerobic activity.

Burn off the supply of excess fat fuel and you've solved one of the problems—a big one, pardon the pun!

MOVE

Which aerobic exercise burns the most calories?

Who knows?

It all depends on the fitness of the person doing the exercise, the level of intensity of the workout, and how much lean muscle mass the person has.

What makes more of a difference than what movement you are doing is the way you are doing it.

Are you moving within your fitness level, increasing and decreasing levels of intensity as you go?

Are you using correct form and working in a focused way?

Consistency is very important when you are talking about effective fat burning—and by the way, that *is* what we're talking about, not burning calories.

Fat.

It's fat that's the issue here.

A very, very unfit beginner, using correct form, walking, focusing, doing it six days a week over a long period of time, can be 10 times more effective a fat-burner than someone who goes out and beats the heck out of herself working outside her fitness level a couple of times a week using all of the latest technology and looking like a superfit hero. . . .

MOVE

What does exercise do to my metabolism?

Increases it.

Makes it function more efficiently.

Gives it the help it needs to do its job for you.

There are two things that slow down or damage a metabolic rate—dieting and lack of exercising.

There are two things that increase and help heal a slow metabolic rate—guess what they are?

Exercise and fuel—food. It's simple when you give your body what it needs to function—it functions beautifully.

Even when we abuse the heck out of it, it keeps right on going. . . .

(I know, I know, just like the Energizer bunny— pardon me, I couldn't resist anything that obvious!)

My life will never be the same again. I finally know that I'm not crazy. I have hope.
—S.N., Washington

MOVE

Do I need to eat before I exercise?

It depends.

Do you like to eat before you exercise? Are you hungry just before you exercise? Do you get nauseated if you eat, then exercise?

Whether to eat a small meal, a light snack—bagel, bread?—or big meal depends on you: your schedule, what type of exercise you are about to do, and what works best for you. You don't NEED to do anything other than listen to your own body and do what feels right.

I don't like to eat before my workout, if I'm working out in the morning, but there's nothing better than a huge lunch and then three or four hours later an all-out workout. WOW, big fun.

There are no rules or regulations. What works for you?

Since it's me you're asking, my answer is: Whatever works for you and whatever gives you the energy you need to focus, work within your fitness level, and get the most out of your workout.

MOVE

Wouldn't it be best to lose the weight, then start exercising to tone up?

THIS IS IT. Staring right at me is the confusion and bad information we've all gotten from the diet industry and the likes of 'em.

You can't burn the body fat without the exercise. . . .

The cardio-endurance can't build without the exercise.

The strength and muscle tone can't build without the exercise.

The oxygen ain't going to get into every cell and every muscle of your body without the exercise. . . .

And if you *are* dieting, you shouldn't be exercising at all.

Think about it—if you are not putting in enough fuel to get through the day, how can you require your body to burn extra fuel by adding exercise to your list of bodily demands without giving it the fuel it needs?

So let's switch this question around. Shouldn't I start exercising within my fitness level (I added that) so that I can lose the extra body fat (I added that too) and get strong and physically fit?

YES.

There, we fixed it. I feel better now.

MOVE

I lead a really active life: three kids, busy job, husband, volunteer work. It seems like I'm up and moving all the time. Do I really need an exercise program?

Busy is one thing.

Exercise is another.

In taking care of all those people, you've left someone out. YOU.

Your body needs exercise to be well, and if you are not well, it sounds like a lot of people won't get their needs met.

Take the time—it's only a few minutes a day, and you'll have the energy to stay busy for a long, long time.

> *Today, if you're not confused, you're not thinking clearly.*
> —Irene Paul

MOVE

How often do I need to exercise?

If you do an aerobic activity three times a week, you maintain what you've got. That's wonderful if what you've got is what you want.

But if you've got some fat to burn and some cardio-endurance to increase, doing an aerobic activity five or six times a week is the deal.

It's simple. In the beginning, you have to make the internal changes by moving within your fitness level (so it's never torture, only pure, oxygenated pleasure) five or six times a week, in order to make the external permanent. Then you maintain it all by working out three times a week.

But you know what? When you get strong and healthy and your body is feeling better than it has in years, you're gonna look at that three-day-a-week maintenance program and laugh—

Movement when it's done properly is heaven, and you're gonna want that slice of heaven in your life daily. . . .

Wait and see!

You don't have to be afraid of change. Don't worry about what's been taken away. Just look to see what's been added.
                                                        —Jackie Greer

MOVE

I have a really busy job and can't find the time to exercise during the week. Can I just do a couple of long workouts on the weekend instead of spacing it out throughout the week?

No! Stop! Don't do it!

You are setting yourself up for burnout, injury, and all kinds of things. An unfit body can't take a couple of hours of working out twice a week if you don't do anything all week long.

A busy schedule is something I can really understand, believe me. I have an ex-husband, a current husband, two kids, and a very, very full-time job, but I'm telling you the truth when I say that if you are beating the heck out of yourself twice a week you are not doing much of anything.

Come on, you can find 30 minutes a day. Early morning or late evening walk? Something to get some oxygen into your body four times a week? Make the weekend two of your 30–45-minute aerobic workouts and then all you have to do is find 30 minutes twice during the week.

Nobody understands busy like I do—but there's no better time investment like those 30 minutes.

MOVE

How long do I need to exercise?

That depends on what you want to accomplish.

If it's the next Ironman Triathlon you want to get ready for, I think it's about 10 hours a day of training. The New York City Marathon, a couple of hours a day at least.

If what you want to do is burn some fat, increase muscular strength and cardio-endurance, then you can do an aerobic activity for 30 minutes or more—no more than an hour—more than three times a week, and you're set.

Building your cardio-endurance and strength isn't difficult at all—and burning some fat is just a matter of cutting back on the amount you're putting in and burning the extra off.

I feel so much better about myself. I don't care if my thighs are rubbing together right now—one day they won't. And you better believe on that day I'm going to throw the biggest party ever.

—M.M., California

MOVE

Can I exercise too much?

In a big way. You can do anything too much. I've been on a 36-year journey and have proven that over and over again.

It's not how often you exercise that counts, it's making your time count while you are exercising that's important. If you are moving with control, resistance, extension, and modifying within your fitness level, building from one fitness level to the next—then, you're doing something good.

If you are compulsively exercising seven days a week, working way beyond your fitness level not using correct form—what are you doing?

Sure, you can exercise too much, but you won't need to once you learn how to do it right—you'll be too busy living to spend all day in the gym.

We teach what we learn and the cycle goes on.
—Joan L. Curcio

MOVE

I've always been overweight and I have never exercised. What is something easy and inexpensive that I can do?

Walking within your fitness level in oxygen for 30 minutes and breathe, breathe, breathe, breathe. . . . .
It's inexpensive, it's easy—and it works.

Don't wait for your ship to come in and feel angry and cheated when it doesn't. Get going with something small.

—Irene Kassorla

MOVE

***I'm really unfit, and I can't make it through a
whole hour of exercising, or even 30 minutes.
What do I do?***

Can't make it through at what level?

Who's leading you?

What are you doing as your aerobic exercise, and
at what intensity?

You *can* make it through 30 minutes of movement
if you decrease your level of intensity. Walking
around the block 10 times at 260 pounds was impossible for me if I tried to walk fast, or jog, but when I
slowed down to a snail's pace—which is what my
fitness level was—it was possible.

The walking at a snail's pace for 30 minutes is
what built the cardio-endurance, started to burn
some of the fat, and began to increase the muscular
strength enough for me to increase the level of intensity.

So—decrease your level of intensity and start to
build your fitness level.

MOVE

What do you mean by modification?

Well, it's something I haven't learned how to do, except in exercising. Look at my hair—not exactly a modified 'do, wouldn't you say?

But when it comes to exercise, I'll tell you exactly what it means because I do it every time I move.

To modify is to move within your fitness level, physical considerations, fatigue level, hormone level, fight-with-your-husband-level—whatever your level is that you need to work with every time you exercise.

Instead of driving through your workout, hating every minute, stay in oxygen, work at your fitness level—modification is the only way to do that—increasing and decreasing your level of intensity as you go, and getting fit.

All exercise can be modified by slowing the pace, dropping your arms, marching in place if you're out of breath. Levels of intensity can be increased or decreased according to your fitness level, and that makes fitness for everyone, which is the way it should be.

You'll be modifying for the rest of your wonderfully fit life.

MOVE

I have to start modifying two minutes into my workout. Will I ever get stronger?

YES.

Believe me, yes, yes, yes, yes—

If your exercising is consistent.

It makes no difference at all how unfit you are or that you have to modify immediately. All that means is that you are a muscular and cardio weenie—so what?

All the more reason to build some muscle strength and cardio-endurance.

The hardest part about beginning to exercise is facing how unfit you are.

Just know you can absolutely go from being a cardio weenie to whatever you want to be.

I couldn't walk around the block without feeling like I was going to die—so I slowed down, faced the fact that I was as unfit as they come, and started slowly, consistently, to build to the level I have now.

It was easy, enjoyable, and the best investment I ever made.

YES, you can and will be strong and healthy again. Keep going.

It is no sin to attempt and fail. The only sin is not to make the attempt.

—SuEllen Fried

MOVE

On days when I don't seem to have much energy and I can't work out as hard, am I still burning fat?

MODIFICATION.

Here it is. Sure—you're doing something, you're exercising, and that's great. You are going to have different energy levels for a million different reasons.

Each workout is about what you are doing, your fitness level, and what you are trying to accomplish *at the time.*

The definition of a good workout is no longer a killer-hard workout.

A good workout is about whether you were in oxygen, whether you modified (increasing and decreasing your level of intensity), used correct form, focused, enjoyed, burned fat, increased strength and cardio-endurance, worked toward your fitness goal. . . .

Did your workout relieve stress and give you the energy you needed?

Did it feel good?

A good workout? *You* define that, not some incorrect industry standard.

MOVE

***Do I have to beat myself up to burn fat? What
about the old saying, "No pain, no gain"?***

The dumbest saying on earth.

An industry was built on that saying and an industry will die on that saying, unless they learn to teach modification and correct movement, because you guys are getting way too smart to fall for that crap anymore.

No pain, no gain? Absolutely not—as a matter of fact, beating yourself up is the worst thing you can do if you want to stick to any kind of exercise. I mean, think about it: Who would volunteer for an hour of torture a day and do it for any length of time?

It is better to work at a lower level of intensity for a longer period of time than it is to get in there and beat the hell out of yourself for a few sessions each week.

The way to get lean, strong, and healthy is to work at a lower level of intensity, *consistently,* for a decent period of time—and ENJOY.

*We must remember that one determined person can
make a significant difference, and that a small
group of determined people can change the course
of history.*
—Sonia Johnson

MOVE

I hate exercise. Is it really important, or can I just eat less?

Eating less will only give you less energy.

Eating less fat is important whether you are exercising or not.

I don't believe it's exercise you hate.

Maybe you hate aerobic classes—who could blame you for that?

Perhaps jogging's not your deal—who could blame you there either?

But you hate all forms of moving for 30 minutes or more in oxygen?

Come on, a nice walk to get some oxygen and reconnect with your body?

If you want to be healthy and have energy, exercise is important.

Having oxygen, cardio-endurance, and lean muscle mass keeps you fit, well, looking and feeling good—and exercise is what that's all about. So think beyond just losing weight, and find anything you like doing for 30 minutes in oxygen.

MOVE

I'm very hungry after exercising. Is it okay to eat?

Yeah, yeah, yeah—that's not the beginning of a Beatles song, it's the answer to the question.

Yeah, yeah, yeah, it's okay to eat when you're hungry, *especially* when you've been exercising.

You're hungry because your body needs fuel.

You're hungry because your body is developing lean muscle mass.

You're hungry because your machine is functioning.

The issue is no longer if it's okay to eat, it's what you're eating. Did you just work out and sit down to a bucket full of fried chicken, or are you eating high-quality, high-volume, low-fat, wonderful food? That's the most important deal.

Which is it?

Eating is okay. Eating is a positive thing. WOW.
—M.B.D., New Jersey

MOVE

I get very thirsty when I exercise. Is it okay to stop to get some water?

If you are thirsty, drink.

You should drink when you are thirsty.

Try not to get to the point of dehydration. Drink when you need it, rehydrate your sweating body—and keep going!

MOVE

Do I need to be sweating to be burning fat?

You need to be in oxygen, with an elevated heart rate for 30 minutes or more to be burning fat.

Sweating is a very personal thing. Some people sweat buckets. Some people sweat sweetly.

It's not mandatory that you pour buckets of sweat to be burning fat, but if your heart is elevated and you are moving for more than 30 minutes, you are probably going to break some kind of sweat.

I am now more knowledgeable, informed, and empowered with personal choice and control. I know you didn't do this, but you graciously gave me the tool to help myself to become what I deserve: LEAN, STRONG, AND HEALTHY.
— M.R., Indiana

MOVE

I've been walking for 30 minutes five days a week for two months. Do I need to start increasing how far or how long I walk?

CONGRATULATIONS!
YIPPEE, ANOTHER PERSON GETTING FIT. Good for you.

You don't need to walk further. You need to increase your level of intensity.

Are you filing your nails and making your grocery list while you are walking? You don't need to walk further, but with a higher level of intensity to challenge your body and take it to a new level of fitness. Try adding some arms pressing up and down while you walk—raising arms above your head adds intensity immediately.

How about some stairs? Walk that track and every 10 or 15 minutes walk up the stadium stairs. No stadium nearby? How about a hill? Adding elevation works wonders for your heart rate.

You don't even need to go outside to find the hill, just add some elevation on your treadmill.

Increasing your level of intensity during your 30–45 minutes of aerobic activity is the answer to building the next fitness level. You'll be increasing beyond your wildest dreams as you get fit.

Don't go further, go deeper, lift higher, press stronger, concentrate more—and be well.

MOVE

What does stretching do for me? It seems like such a waste of time.

Lengthens and stretches muscles that are contracted and tight.

Increases flexibility.

Good flexibility increases range of motion.

Works toward the prevention of injury.

Feels so good you could lie down and never get up at the end of a challenging workout.

Gives you a minute in the middle of a life with not many minutes to yourself.

Waste of time? Not at all.

It's time very well spent!

MOVE

Is it better to stretch when I start my workout, or after I finish?

The way to warm up a muscle is to get blood and oxygen to the muscle. The best way to do that is to move.

Slowly.

Start moving and breathing. Get your blood pumping and your muscles warm, then pick up the pace for your 30 minutes in aerobic activity.

Then do the same thing to cool down—slow the pace for a few minutes until you have finished.

Great warmup, great workout, great cooldown.

Then, when the muscles have been worked, are warm, have plenty of blood and oxygen flowing through . . .

When you have been aerobic for 30 minutes . . .

It's a wonderful time to stretch your muscles and your mind.

Slow, calm, controlled stretching. Lifting and pressing. Perfect form. Meditative.

STRRRRRRREEEEEEETTTTTCCCCCHHHHH.

It's the best.

Happiness is good health and a bad memory.
—Ingrid Bergman

MOVE

I've just started exercising, and I'm finding that the next morning I'm very sore. Am I doing something wrong?

Let me start with a big salute to you—

YOU ARE GIVING YOURSELF THE BEST GIFT YOU CAN GIVE—WELLNESS. BLARE THE TRUMPETS, THIS LADY IS GETTING FIT!

Now, let me answer your question.

There's sore, and then there's SORE.

Sore so you can't walk isn't good. That means you need to decrease your level of intensity and work within your fitness level, which may be a very, very beginning one.

Then there's sore that means muscles that haven't been used in 15 years have just had a bit of a wake-up call. That's a good kind of sore. That happens at every level of getting fit. I recently tried a yoga class, thinking, "What's this? Who couldn't do this stuff? Bending and twisting—so what?"

Well, you want sore. . . . I woke up the next day feeling muscles that I don't think are even listed in physiology books. I have *never*—

That was a good kind of sore, but I didn't appreciate it for a couple of days. . . .

MOVE

If I'm really sore from a workout, should I not exercise the next day?

The "calf-locking" sore means you didn't work within your fitness level, didn't modify. That kind of sore needs to spend some time recovering and learning modification so that you never end up like that again.

The "haven't-used-your-muscles-in-20-years" kind of sore is a good kind of sore and begins to go away as your muscles get stronger and used to being used. If that's the kind of sore you're talking about, then yes, exercise again the next day, working within your "sore" level. Do a longer warmup.

Keep working toward getting lean, strong, and healthy—and not sore.

More important to me than the weight loss, which seemed effortless, is the feeling of health and well-being.

—L.S., New York

MOVE

***Which is more important when I exercise,
using my arms and upper body or my legs? I
can't seem to do them both.***

Great question, because there are so many people
who don't have the coordination to move arms and
legs together, and you don't have a chance in hell of
keeping up in most aerobics classes. (Hey, if you
aren't a wanna-be professional dancer, you don't
have a chance in most of them.)

Both your arms and your legs do a lot to keep your
heart rate up. So you can use either/or. Pressing
your arms over your head will increase your cardio
within minutes. So will using larger muscle
groups—legs!

So you have a choice. Whatever works for you.
Whatever feels the most comfortable, and whatever
move works within your coordination level. Drop the
arms anytime and keep the legwork going, or
switch—march in place and do the arms.

Options aplenty!

MOVE

What do you mean by form and resistance?

Correct form is the way a movement is done. Correct form will get you the most out of your movement, help prevent injury, and get you to the next fitness level fastest.

You can·walk, body schlepped over, stomach hanging, and dragging along, or you can WALK!

Try this: body lifted, shoulders pressed down, no tension in the neck, and then resist while you walk. Instead of dangling or swinging your arms by your side, try pressing them through mud. . . . That's it, think mud, quicksand, water— and add resistance to your press and pull.

Arms, legs, body resisting while you are walking in correct form, always within your fitness level, never out of breath, increasing and decreasing your level of intensity as you go, and BAMMO, you've got a very different walk.

You've got a walk that's going to burn fat, increase your endurance, build strength, and get you fit.

Who would have thought we could modify? I'm modifying on my treadmill and feel like I've been resurrected from the dead. The pain, the depression, the humiliation—it's all lifting. I can say that and mean it.
—F.R., Louisiana

MOVE

I have no energy in the morning to exercise, but it's the only time I have to work out. What can I do?

Start moving so that you have energy.

Without exercise, high-quality low-fat fuel, and some strength, you're not gong to have energy.

Without energy you can't live—well, you can, but it doesn't feel good to live with no energy. I've done it.

Waking up every day with a foundation of wellness and the energy you need to get out of bed and function is so much better.

Start slow, at a low level of intensity, and keep it up. Within a few days, you'll have the energy you need to keep going, and before you know it, you'll be bounding out of bed and feeling great.

Ready to start your morning exercise.

Life begets life. Energy creates energy. It is by spending oneself that one becomes rich.
—Sarah Bernhardt

MOVE

Where do I find the energy to exercise after working all day?

In high-quality fuel.

In making sure you are getting enough calories during the day.

In building a foundation of wellness that gives you more energy than you could ever imagine, and keeps you going after 5 P.M.

And in knowing that the energy comes from the movement, and that if you *do* move, you'll feel 10 times better than if you don't.

I know sometimes it feels like you just can't do it, but I've never heard anyone leave an exercise class saying, "I wish I hadn't done that." I've heard and said thousands of times, "Wow, I'm sure glad I did that. I feel so much better."

My God, my God, my God! I've just finished the first time ever of working out for one hour. No one could have told me I could do it until your video. I've never worked out for one hour before at anything. I modified.

—N.D., Texas

MOVE

Does exercise really reduce stress?

In a big, big, big, big way.

Having the option of going for a walk, jog, row, hike, bike—rather than stewing in whatever's stressing you out—is a blessing.

While you are exercising, the oxygen pumping through your body, your muscles working, your body sweating out the toxins, your brain releasing endorphins left, right, and center—it all works together to make you feel a whole lot better at the end of a good workout.

Here is what I hear after a good workout, "Gosh, I feel so much better—I'm ready to go home and face the family."

Or, "Let's keep going—I have more strength than I've had all day."

Or, "Why didn't I think of this earlier? I'm so glad I did it. I feel great!"

That's what stress reduction sounds like.

To move freely, you must be deeply rooted.
                                    —Bella Lewitzky

MOVE

Will exercise help me sleep?

That depends on what your sleeping problem is, but I'll tell you something.

After a full, productive day, and then a strong, sweating-bullets kind of workout (always within your fitness level), a hot bath, and a cozy bed—it's coma time for me.

I didn't sleep well when I was 260 pounds. I was uncomfortable, always tired without doing anything, and nighttime was a very difficult time for me.

It was when the babies were asleep and I'd be alone with my deepest fear—would I ever to able to break this cycle, and look and feel better? Another diet failed that day, more eating that night?

Fear, anger, shame, pain—all surfaced at night, and it interfered with a lot of things in my life. Sleep was just one of them.

Try getting well, and see if it helps your particular sleeping problem.

It's not gonna do any harm, and it might help.

MOVE

I have two small babies and no help around the house. What can I do to exercise?

Hi, fellow mom with two babies and no help.

First, I want to tell you that the job you are doing is the hardest job on earth and you deserve a statue erected in your honor along with every other mom in this country raising babies with no help.

Time is very valuable and hard to find when you are raising two small babies. Paying a babysitter is fine if you can afford it and if you can find one who isn't a lunatic, but the bottom line is that you need to be able to do something at home or with the kids—and there *are* options.

Home videos are good because you can take a class in your living room while the kids are playing or sleeping. Of course, I'd recommend mine—you can strength train and do aerobics with us—but whichever one works for you, try it.

Then there's walking. A great activity with the kids, and even on the lousiest weather days, there's always the mall. Take the kids in the stroller and walk through the mall at an aerobic pace—you'll burn some fat. If the kids swim, there's always swimming. They can play and you can get some laps in.

Raise wonderful, responsible children and get yourself fit—and you've done the world and yourself a favor.

MOVE

I'm over 65. Do I need to do some kind of special workout?

Special because *you* are special.

Not any different than what all of us have to do to burn fat—increase muscular strength and cardio-endurance.

One thing that is very important as you get older is building strength. There are a lot of weight-lifting seniors out there now that fitness is for everyone.

So—I say we should add a senior category to the Mr. and Ms. America weight-lifting competitions right away.

I'm 50 years old, have four children, three grandchildren, and have been married for 32 years to the same man. I feel that I've been dead for the past 20 years. I weight 180 and hate my body image. As of today I have taken the first step to change my life. I have no idea where that will eventually take me but I'm excited about it.

—R.G., Canada

MOVE

I'm in a wheelchair. What exercises can I do?

Upper body anything—if you can move your upper body.

Abdominal work, if you have feeling and control of your abdominal wall.

Arms, if that's possible.

I went to the Dallas Rehab Center recently with some TV cameras and spoke to a wonderful group of people in wheelchairs. What I found was that people who are physically challenged—the 90s politically correct term for handicapped (I know, 'cause I asked)—have the exact same needs and reasons for exercise that everybody does.

Here's what I heard:

"I want to regain control over my life."

"My upper body aches. I want strength back."

"I'm tired and want more energy."

"After my second baby, I don't like the way I look and feel. It's time to get back into shape."

It's funny—when you can't see the chair and you just hear the needs, you see how similar we all are.

MOVE

I have back problems that prevent me from doing aerobic classes. Is there something else I can do?

There's something you *have* to do.

You *have* to do an aerobic activity if you want to burn fat. But that has very little to do with aerobic classes.

Think:

Nonimpact
Noninvasive
Not jolting

Think:

Stationary equipment (bike, treadmill)
Swimming
Walking

Do the aerobic activity so that you burn the excess fat, especially the fat on your stomach pulling on your back.

Then build some strength to support your weakened back. Add flexibility and stretching to relax.

Ask your doctor what happens when you add more fat to your stomach, lose more muscular strength, and get weaker.

MOVE

Some days my arthritis is so bad I can't use my arms to exercise. Should I just skip exercise that day?

Well, you can exercise and not use your arms.

Those big leg muscles can send your heart rate through the roof—use them if you can.

Get your cardio up, burn the fat, and get that oxygen to your joints.

If it's just a question of not using your arms, you're okay—because you have a choice.

MOVE

Should I exercise when I'm sick?

How sick are we talking here?

If you're heaving every few minutes, I wouldn't suggest exercise, but if you are just not feeling well, a little tired and out of sorts, then get a little oxygen working at the level of intensity that feels right, and see how you feel.

Maybe some oxygen will make you feel better. Use your common sense and listen to your body.

Exercise can't hurt you if you do it properly. Not exercising can.

MOVE

I was ill last week and couldn't work out. Will I be starting all over again?

That depends on what your fitness level was before you got sick.

Was this the first time you'd worked out in years? Then, yeah, you probably will be starting over again.

Were you already very physically fit? If so, then no, you simply lost a couple of days of exercise.

You see, when your body has a foundation of wellness, it functions at a different level than a body that is overfat, unfit, and lacking strength.

So, if that was your first week, start again—you didn't lose anything.

Feel good again and work out.

You may have to fight a battle more than once to win.
                                    —Margaret Thatcher

MOVE

What special exercises can I do to get rid of cellulite?

Jogging to the office of anyone who's telling you that cellulite is anything other than fat—and bashing them over the head!

That's a good cellulite exercise.

Cellulite is nothing more than fat, and there's only one way to get rid of fat—you've got to burn it off.

MOVE

You say to lift my abdominal muscle, but I can't feel anything. What do you mean?

You can't feel what you don't have. There may be no abdominal strength yet.

It took me a couple of months before I could feel that lift too.

Don't worry if you can't feel it right away.

Building a strong lower, middle, and upper abdominal wall takes time.

You will feel it once it's stronger and not covered with fat.

All adventures, especially into new territory, are scary.

—Sally Ride

MOVE

My husband says, the faster I run, the more effective it is—and the faster I'll lose weight.

Hub, what happens if you are not fit enough to run? Then what the heck are you supposed to do?

What happens if you are so unfit that running fast would kill you?

NO.

It is much more effective to move at a slower pace for a longer period of time and build to different levels than it is to beat the hell out of yourself.

Running faster to get faster results as the husband suggests does two things.

It sets you up for death or injury, depending on how unfit you are, *and* failure. You are absolutely not going to maintain your new beat-the-hell-out-of-yourself lifestyle for any length of time because nobody gets up and looks forward to a voluntary beating—so it won't last.

You should tell your husband what millions of women have been telling their husbands for centuries:

Slow down.

It's the quality, not the quantity.

It's better to go slowly for a long period of time than to give it all in seconds. . . . .

You know what I'm talking about!

MOVE

I can tell I'm looking leaner around my neck and upper body, but nothing seems to be moving on the bottom half! How can I make the fat come off my hips?

I love you—this is a great question!

Here's how you can make the fat come off your hips—by doing the exact same thing you've been doing to make it come off your neck and upper body.

The largest supply is the last to go—take my word for it—but it goes. It goes in a big way, and when it does, it's glorious.

Here's what happened to me. First, just like you, I saw a collarbone. My chest and arms started to look lean, then a rib here and there, then a waist popped up or in out of nowhere, and then the stomach.

The stomach was my most hated area. The hanging fat drove me nuts. Everything else was looking really good and my stomach still hung. But I kept going. Doing the same thing I'm suggesting you do.

You are losing body fat. You are getting leaner. So keep going, and guess what's going to happen?

It's gonna burn. The largest supply is the last to go, so forget about it, just keep getting lean, strong, and healthy, and feeling better than you have in years.

LET IT BURN.

MOVE

Is strength training more important than aerobic exercise?

That depends on what you're trying to accomplish.

Are you trying to build cardio-conditioning? If so, a dumbbell ain't going to do you much good.

Are you trying to get some energy and pump some oxygen through your body? A walk and three sets of 10 are both going to do that.

Are you trying to burn tons of fat? Then doing both will get you leaner faster.

It all works together—and it also stands alone, depending on what you want from your workout.

I'm very strong-willed and in control of most areas of my life. By feeling out of control with my weight, I was doubting myself in all other areas. I'm gaining my confidence back.

—H.D., Oregon

MOVE

Do I do strength training every day?

Upper and lower body and abdominal strength training can be done every day.

But if you are building lean muscle mass with heavy reps—otherwise known as body building—your upper and lower body needs a day of rest and recovery between workouts.

Your abdominals can be worked every day.

Building strength and endurance sure feels good—I just did it an hour ago.

If I'm too strong for some people, that's their problem.
—Glenda Jackson

MOVE

Will I build bulky muscles if I use weights?

If it's bulk you are worried about—worry about fat.

One pound of muscle and one pound of fat weight the same.

But that one pound of fat takes up five times the volume in the human body. It's fat that's bulky. Building lean muscle mass will help you burn some of that bulky fat off.

Here's the deal: fat is bulky; muscle tissue is busy, busy, busy burning fat.

So don't worry, pick up the dumbbell.

I can now do the military press—three sets of 10 with 1½-pound weights. When I started, I could barely do 10 without weights. I am actually developing muscular strength now where there wasn't any.

—B.B., California

MOVE

I'm really obese. If I do strength training, is it going to make me bigger?

NO.

Do you know what those people in the bodybuilding magazines have to do to get that God-awful look? (In all due respect, it's the ugliest thing I've ever seen.) To achieve it they have to lift hundreds of pounds of weights, be unbelievably disciplined with diet and training, and work like hell to build the bulk necessary to look like that.

If you are obese, start lifting weights right away, along with your aerobic activity, because muscle is metabolically the most active tissue in the body. Active means fuel-burning, fuel-burning means *fat*-burning, and fat-burning means a leaner you. . . .

MOVE

I'm in good shape except for the saddlebags on my thighs. What are some good exercises to trim down?

Those saddlebags are fat bags.

Check your body fat percentage and burn off what you don't want.

You may be in a size 6 pair of jeans and still have an unhealthy percent of body fat with saddlebags aplenty. There's only one way to get them off your thighs—

Burn, baby, burn.

MOVE

*What about those arm flaps—
can anything help?*

That stuff that hangs underneath our arms—don't you love it? Isn't it the worst when you point to give someone directions and your arm wiggles? How about sleeveless dresses—when was the last time you wore one?

Well, believe me—there's an answer, and it's the same answer to the fat that's hanging from anywhere . . . your stomach, your thighs.

You've got to burn it off, and you can—from anywhere. Thirty minutes of aerobic activity more than three times a week will burn that fat from under your arms and everywhere else. Think about that extra fat as the fuel your body is going to start using the minute you cut back on the fat you are taking in and start moving within your fitness level to burn it off.

Don't think of it as a genetic inheritance. That flab is extra fuel and you've got to use it up, burn it off, to lose it forever.

MOVE

Do those dopey-looking face exercises really do anything?

Yeah, they make you look like a lunatic.

But who knows? Your face has muscles in it, movement strengthens muscles, and I suppose it could help. However, it's not a big fat-burner . . . and I'd suggest you do it only in the privacy of your own home.

MOVE

Will sit-ups make the fat around my middle go away?

Nope.

No chance.

But aerobic activity will burn the fat from your stomach and everywhere else on your body, and the sit-ups you are going to do along with your aerobic activity will increase the strength in your abdominal wall . . .

Which will help support your lower back . . .

Give you that great strong stomach look when the fat burns off . . .

And make you feel fabulous, because a strong stomach is the center of a strong body.

That fat will burn and those muscles will get strong.

Do both.

I am now on my way to getting healthy and I feel so good. I have a lot of hope for a great future.
— D.D., Washington

MOVE

What's the best way, aside from surgery, to flatten your stomach?

Let's start with the fact that surgery *isn't* the best way to flatten your stomach—take it from me, I've had a tummy tuck. (I had the surgery *after* I got lean, strong, and healthy.)

If you have lots of fat hanging from your stomach, surgery isn't going to solve the problem. Sure, right after the nips and the tuck, your stomach will be flatter, but you'll gain it back unless you deal with . . . you guessed it, burning the fat, increasing the muscle strength underneath the fat. Then have the tummy tuck if you want it.

The best way to flatten your stomach is to do aerobic activity to burn the fat—from your stomach and everywhere else—and include abdominal exercises (yes, the infamous sit-ups and crunches) to increase the strength in the muscles underneath.

If there was any cosmetic surgery on earth that could burn 133 pounds, increase lean muscle mass and strength, and build cardio-endurance, then count me in. I'd be the first in line and I'd recommend it to the world.

There isn't.

After you get lean, strong, and healthy, nip and tuck anything you want.

MOVE

I keep hearing about cross-training. What is it, and do I need to be doing it?

Cross-training is fun and any fitness level can do it, and you should be doing it.

Cross-training means that one day you walk, the next day you bike, then throw in a little strength training, and maybe top off your workout week with a kick-boxing lesson. . . . Oh, sure, something most of us are interested in!

Cross-train different muscle groups. Cross-train different levels of concentration and challenge. Cross-train your interests—and cross-train your fat-burning.

There's nothing fancy about it, nothing difficult, and you don't need special equipment or a personal trainer.

Think about what you enjoy doing, mix it all up, and enjoy!

MOVE

Exercise tapes and classes always confuse me. I have two left feet. Does it do me any good to try and keep up?

No.

Stop trying to keep up.

Most of us spend so much time trying to figure out the next step that we end up starting and stopping and standing there in confusion.

Turn the video off and do an aerobic activity that doesn't require you to dance your way through it.

You do not have to be brilliantly coordinated to burn fat.

You simply have to burn it in oxygen, not in choreography.

Rowing.

Swimming.

Bike riding.

Walking.

It's your choice.

Don't wait for leaders; do it alone, person to person.
                                    —Mother Teresa

MOVE

Is swimming a good form of exercise for burning fat?

Swimming is an excellent aerobic exercise, if it's in oxygen for 30 minutes or more, and with an elevated heart rate—that means fat-burning.

But do me a favor, if you're a man reading this and getting ready to go for a swim. Please spare us—don't wear one of those little speedy weedy bathing suits, unless you're an Olympic athlete. Otherwise you probably look really goofy.

Put on a proper suit, go for a swim, and burn that fat.

MOVE

What do you think about water aerobics?

If it's done right, it's a wonderful form of aerobic activity.

Water provides great resistance and is very effective to work with or against as the case may be. Most people have no idea how difficult using water is until they try exercising in it.

Water aerobics is a fun, diverse, and challenging workout, and offers many advantages to people dealing with special physical considerations *and* to the physically fit.

Just remember, if you are outside, wear a hat—my friend just had a huge skin cancer taken from her face because of too much sun!

Wear a hat and burn some fat—hey, there's a saying for your water aerobics class.

Wear a hat and burn some fat.

I like it!

MOVE

My husband says golf is good exercise. Is that true?

Golfers—aren't they a breed unto themselves?

Golf involves walking, unless you take a cart.

Golf involves precision, planning, definitely a certain disposition—can you see me golfing?

NEVER.

Hate to break it to the husband, but golf is not aerobic and it's not up there on the ten-best-ways-to-burn-fat exercise list.

Have a look at some of the guys playing. Great physical specimens?

Sometimes I wonder if men and women really suit each other. Perhaps they should live next door and just visit now and then.
—Katharine Hepburn

MOVE

Is going out dancing with my husband good exercise?

It's great—if you dance for 30 to 45 minutes with an elevated heart rate and without stopping.

I'm not sure that combining your evening out with the husband and your aerobic workout is such a great idea, but if dancing, sweating, and burning fat can be done all at once and it's what you want to do, then go for it.

MOVE

What do you think of those cross-country ski machines?

Cross-country skiing is a fabulous aerobic exercise; those cross-country skiing machines are a different story. Have you ever tried one? Before you buy—try (kind of poetic, don't you think?). Get on one, put that band that some of them have around your waist, hang on to the handles, and get ready—

Get ready to spend your whole workout trying to stay on the damn thing! If you find a cross-country ski machine that is easy to use, let me know—I'd like to try it. Every one that I've tried has been awkward and difficult to manage. The bottom line for you and your fitness level is, why do it when walking is a great aerobic activity? Why spend the money, where are you going to store it (some of them are huge!), and why is it necessary?

It's not the piece of equipment that's going to change your body. There's no special answer in chrome and steel, only in changing the way you look and feel forever by moving in oxygen for 30 minutes or more, increasing lean muscle mass, and increasing cardio-endurance and strength. Bingo. So what do I think of them? Not much.

MOVE

I like to go shopping at the mall. Isn't this good exercise?

Shopping as exercise? Absolutely not!

Mall walking can be a good aerobic exercise, not the shopping.

How about going 45 minutes early? Do your mall walk and then shop. That way, you can get both activities in.

MOVE

Is pushing a baby stroller around the block exercise?

Yep, for 30 minutes in oxygen with an elevated heart rate.

Good exercise.

Fat-burning exercise.

Sure is.

The phrase "working mother" is redundant.
                                    —Jane Sellman

MOVE

Does housework count as exercise?

Housework counts for a lot. Organization, management, creating a loving, peaceful environment.... Am I starting to sound like a meditation book? Well, this isn't—it's a fitness book, and the fitness answer to the question is no, housework is not exercise unless you vacuum for 30 minutes, with an elevated heart rate, and include a warmup and cooldown (in which case you wouldn't need to vacuum, you might as well work out).

MOVE

Do I really have to work out every day?

Absolutely not! Once your body is internally fit—some lean muscle mass, a healthy percent body fat, strong heart and lungs—then all you need is maintenance—three or four aerobic workouts a week—and you can maintain your aerobic fitness level.

But let me ask you something. Are you trying to burn tons of fat? Have you yet to build any lean muscle mass? Are you trying to change a very unfit body? If so, you need to do an aerobic activity *at least* four to five times a week to begin to make the internal changes that will get you results—and that will make the external changes permanent.

(Unless, of course, you stop moving and start eating high-fat food—then you and I both know what's going to happen.)

Eating, breathing, and moving within your lifestyle, fitness level, and physical consideration is the only way to change how you look and feel.

MOVE

I'm going on vacation soon. Do you have any suggestions for working out while traveling?

Well, the actual traveling is a little difficult—working out on a plane can be tough!

But once you're there—depending on where you go—you just keep on doing what you've been doing.

Walking?

Jogging?

Aerobic classes?

Stationary bike?

Going to the gym?

The great part about exercising while you're on vacation is that you can add diversity and challenge to your daily workout.

I mean, if you've just flown in from the wheat field to Hawaii, try hiking one of those mountains.

From the south to the north—how about cross-country skiing?

East Coast to West Coast—maybe surfing?

Remember, anything can be modified, so try different things and don't worry about exercising on your vacation—it's a chance to diversify.

MOVE

Can't I just work out and not worry about eating low-fat?

If you don't mind all the other things a high-fat diet does to your body, other than make you fat . . .

Like heart disease?

You can do anything you want, but cutting back on your daily fat intake is about much more than just having lean thighs, although lean thighs are very, very important.

So are your arteries.

I know I have gained nothing if I sacrifice my health to be thinner.

— F.F., Louisiana

MOVE

*I'm so fat I'm too embarrassed to go anywhere
and work out. What can I do?*

Exactly what you did—acknowledge the problem.
Here's what you do. Do something that doesn't
require you to go anywhere and work out. But understand that unless you start the process of burning fat, increasing strength, and getting well, it's
only going to get worse.

Stationary bike.
Video.
Treadmill.
Walking around your neighborhood.
Mall walking—pretend you're shopping and they'll never know!

Anything that works for you that is an aerobic
activity and that doesn't embarrass you.

You can solve the problem, and then strut into any
damn place to work out when you are looking and
feeling the way you want to look and feel—and strut
you will.

*The distance is nothing. It is only the first step
that's difficult.*
—Mme. du Deffand

MOVE

I'm so weak in my arms that I can't lift the weights. How should I start?

By not lifting the weights.

You don't have to lift your arms any more than once if that's all you can do.

How about this? Go for a walk, and once every couple of minutes press your arms up in the air and then press them down. There are two parts to every movement—the lift up and the press down—make them both count. Do it only once. Continue walking. Then do it again.

Do you know what you will be doing? Working within your fitness level and building to the next. As your arms get stronger, you'll be able to lift and press them up and down as many times as you want.

Be patient, be consistent in your exercise, and watch what happens.

Build it—it's the best feeling in the world.

Your arms will get stronger and stronger.

The thing that women have to learn is that nobody gives you power. You just take it.
                                    —Roseanne Arnold

MOVE

I'm so overweight that I'm afraid it's not safe to exercise. What should I do?

Here's what's not safe—*not* to exercise.

So you have to start moving.

Walking at a low level of intensity isn't going to kill you, but if you want to be sure, go to your doctor, get a stress test, and ask him or her if going for a low-intensity walk four times a week in oxygen is going to kill you. . . .

NOT doing it is the thing that's going to kill you.

Be afraid *not* to exercise, and get whatever tests you need to reassure you.

Start moving, please, please, please. . . . .

Slowly.

Properly.

Courage is fear that has said its prayers.
— Dorothy Bernard

MOVE

I don't seem to have enough energy to exercise. What should I do?

Exercise before you get less energy. . . .

Exercise gives you energy immediately if you do it properly. You should walk away from your aerobic activity having more energy than when you started.

That's what getting oxygen into your body does for you.

So when you think exercise, think "walk within oxygen," never getting out of breath.

Then think "breathe," taking that energy-giving oxygen into your body.

Then think "Thank God," because the alternative is having less energy and dying. . . .

Don't do that. Come back to life. Get oxygen.

Three days ago I started moving. Today I woke up and did not dread facing the day.

—M.J., Texas

MOVE

Why do I need to exercise?

This is the greatest question.

I could be friends with this lady.

You don't need to exercise if you don't care about being healthy, physically fit, having energy, or looking and feeling good. . . .

But—if you want to have energy, you've got to have good lean muscle mass and cardio-endurance.

If you don't want wads of fat, you've got to burn it off.

If you want a higher-quality life—because being fit feels a whole lot better than being unfit (take it from me, I've done both)—you have to exercise.

And, if you want one of the best preventive steps you can take against heart disease and many other illnesses, then get fit.

I now eat low-fat, move every day, and I feel wonderful. I'm so motivated because I can see myself getting tighter, I look better in my clothes, and I have so much energy. Last Saturday I was able to wear a pair of shorts that had been really tight—I jumped around the house yelling, "Thank you, Susan!"

—G.G., Texas

LIVE

Happiness is not a state to arrive at—but a manner of traveling.
—Margaret Lee Rumbeck

LIVE

You've got the tools.
   EAT.
   BREATHE.
   MOVE.

You're eating high-volume, low-fat, high-quality food.

You're breathing 100 times a day and filling your body with oxygen.

You're moving more than three times a week for 30 minutes and elevating your heart rate.

You've begun to change your life forever. But maybe you still have a few questions. . . .

LIVE

How do I get started?

By eating, breathing, and moving today. It's the only way. Apply this information to your life and know that the results—energy, reducing body fat, increasing strength and endurance—can save you. It can and will change the way you look and feel.

There's not much that feels as good as getting up every day with a foundation of wellness, with the strength and energy you need to get through the day. Or having the energy to recapture your hopes and dreams.

How did I begin? I just started eating, breathing, and moving.

Stop thinking and just start.

I feel so good about myself already because I really believe that this is going to change how I feel and look.

—P.S., Nevada

LIVE

How fast am I going to lose the weight?

You're not going to lose weight until you reduce your body fat. How fast you lose the excess body fat depends on a couple of things:

- How little fat you are taking in daily.
- The quality and quantity of foods you are eating.
- How consistently you're moving within your fitness level.
- How much lean muscle mass you're building.

If you do what has to be done to get fit, you won't even recognize yourself a couple of months into it—and it only gets better and better.

Get fit, that's where it's at! (Doesn't that sound like a line Julie from *The Mod Squad* would have said? You know what I mean. . . .)

LIVE

If I starve myself for a while and exercise, won't I lose weight fast?

Sure you will.

You'll lose a lot of water, lean muscle mass, and yeah, you'll lose weight—but there's a problem.

You'll gain back what you lost and then some immediately.

You'll also do some damage to your body.

You'll slow down your metabolism.

You'll feel horrible because starvation isn't fun or easy.

You'll look awful because that gaunt, drawn look is gross, no matter how skinny you temporarily get.

Yes, you'll lose weight—but you'll lose a lot more than just weight.

And what you lose, you'll gain back . . . and more.

LIVE

How do I know if this is working?

Your clothes falling off is a good indication.

Feeling strength return that you haven't felt in ages is another one.

How about having energy for the first time in years?

These are all good indications that something good is happening.

My big indication that something fabulous was happening was when my thighs stopped rubbing together. I knew I was on the way to something.

I never dreamed it was what it turned out to be.

You may be surprised. Videotapes, books, TV in your future? You never know.

Just keep going and don't worry about it . . . let the dress sizes drop.

The higher the quality of the fuel, the better the performance.

LIVE

How am I supposed to figure out what I am supposed to weigh?

Supposed to weigh, according to whom? Here's a thought: How about not even thinking about the number on the scale and instead determining what you want—not what you're supposed—to feel like?

How much energy and strength do you want?

What dress size looks and feels right for you?

What percentage of body fat do you want to have?

How fit do you need to be to keep up with your life?

Ask yourself those questions and define your own "supposed to"—it's a much better system and has a whole lot more to do with you and your life than those stupid doctors' charts that we've all been living or dying by over the years.

The ultimate lesson all of us have to learn is unconditional love, which includes not only others but ourselves as well.
— Elizabeth Kubler-Ross

LIVE

How fast can you expect to lose weight?

With the speed of lightning if you are starving yourself, but—as you know—you will also gain it back with the speed of lightning.

Burning body fat, increasing lean muscle mass, and building cardio-endurance is a whole different ball game, and it takes a bit longer than a week or two.

How long depends on a couple of things.

First, your daily fat intake. Is it 15% of your day's eating, or 30%?

Then you've got to consider movement. Moving once a week is going to get you fewer results than moving within your fitness level six days a week. If you throw in a little bit of strength training and get those muscles burning more fuel than you could imagine—WOW!

A real old saying applies here: You get out what you put in. Who said that—Rocky?

LIVE

Why is it so easy to regain the weight I just lost on a diet?

Because your body is starving.

Because diets stink.

Because you have been set up to fail like the other 98% of us who lose the weight and gain it back.

Because your metabolic rate is functioning at a nonexistent level, and the minute you put food into your mouth you are going to gain the weight back.

Because that's the way diets work.

Because if you ever reduce calories and continue to function, you are going to lose water and lean muscle mass, and what you lose in lean muscle mass you regain as fat.

Because diets stink . . . they stink, they stink, they stink, and . . . . . .

THEY DON'T WORK.

Please don't ever diet again as long as you live.

There is a solution to this problem, but diets ain't it.

LIVE

My husband tells me that I'll never be able to lose weight because I've failed on every diet I've tried.

Your husband's right—if you go on another diet, you will fail.

But tell the hub something from me, will you? *YOU* HAVE NOT FAILED.

Everyone who's been on a diet, or at least 98% of us, has gained the weight back. It was not our failure, but the failure of the diet industry.

You, just like me and millions of other women, just did the wrong thing.

Now it's time to do it right.

You *can* burn fat. You *can* build lean muscle mass. And you *can* increase cardio-endurance.

Move from the quicksand of injustice to the solid rock of human dignity.
—Dorothy Haight

LIVE

I'm on a diet and it seems the less I eat, the heavier I get. What's wrong with me?

There isn't a thing in the world wrong with you—other than the fact that you've dieted, or you are dieting right now.

When you starve yourself, your body functions in starvation mode. Brilliant, isn't it? Starve it, and that's how it will have to function.

If you haven't eaten in a couple of months, your body becomes very efficient at storing any fuel that comes along at all. The minute you start to eat anything—large or small (pardon the pun)—you'll start gaining back your weight.

You are NOT a genetic mutation. You are like the other 98% of us who have dieted, lost some weight, and gained it and more back the minute we started eating.

Never fear—the answer is here:

DON'T DIET.

High-volume, low-fat food—eat it to help increase your metabolic rate.

Exercise to help increase your metabolic rate and get your body functioning normally.

Starvation only works if you never eat again, and then it only works until it kills you. So you see, it's a very ineffective method.

LIVE

Why hasn't my doctor told me any of this?

That's a very good question.

One that I asked my doctor—just before I fired him.

LIVE

I've been eating this way for two weeks now and I haven't lost any weight. What's wrong?

NOW—

Anyone who knows me knows what's coming next: BURN THE SCALE. GET RID OF THE DAMN THING. ELIMINATE IT FROM YOUR LIFE. And please, please give your body more than two weeks to begin to function properly. We are not talking losing water and lean muscle mass—that is, instant weight loss. You've done that and you know what happens—it's all going to come back and more.

We are talking getting your body well internally, having your body function at a normal healthy level. Burning some body fat, increasing some lean muscle mass, increasing some cardio-endurance—and getting well. THAT CAN'T BE MEASURED ON YOUR BATHROOM SCALE TWO WEEKS INTO THE PROCESS.

So, my suggestion is, get off the scale and forget about it for a couple of months!

I am certainly not thin yet, but the process is making it through each day knowing I have done what I said I was gong to do—and the weight is coming off.

—N.N., Wyoming

LIVE

Why shouldn't I use the scale? Doesn't it tell me if I'm losing weight?

Guys, guys, help me out here!!!

Anyone who has ever read, seen, or listened to anything I've ever done knows the answer to this one. The scale is a piece of bondage equipment that was probably invented by the same guy who invented pantyhose. . . .

THE SCALE IS OUT!

Shrinking is IN.

Clothes sizes dropping is IN.

Having very little fat on your arms and seeing a strong, well-developed muscle underneath is IN, IN, IN.

The days of weighing yourself every minute of the day are GONE. . . .

Think about it.

Because it never did any good, did it? But it sure has done a lot of harm.

Have a scale-burning party on me!!!!!

LIVE

The weight loss was showing on my scale in the beginning, now it seems to be slowing down. What's wrong?

What's wrong, What's wrong???
You're on the scale, that's what's wrong.

Here's the deal.

When you cut back on your daily fat intake and start moving, your body is gong to tap into your fat supply—the stuff on your thighs, your butt, your arms, and everywhere else—and use the excess as its fat fuel. When that happens, you are going to lose a lot of weight because fat is HEAVY.

Then, when you start building some lean muscle mass you pick up the pace at which your fat-burning machine burns. As you fuel that fat-burning machine with the best fuel and enough of it, those coals keep that fire—your metabolic rate—nice and hot. Sounding like a romance novel? Well, it's not. It's your new body and that body will continue to change, develop, and get well, fit, and healthy.

So don't worry about it. Just eat, breathe, and move your way to a new body and a new life.

LIVE

Is my metabolic rate ruined? I've dieted all my life.

No, not ruined—hurting bad, but not ruined.

We've all dieted, all our lives, and some of us have gone to unbelievable extremes. But I haven't met a metabolic rate yet that doesn't respond to eating, exercising, and a few other basic things that your body needs.

(You'll have to ask your doctor whether there's ever been a recorded metabolism ruined for life from the bashing that we all give our bodies.)

But I'm sure your metabolism will respond to the simple, easy, effective methods of eating, breathing, and moving.

You can rebuild a healthy, well-functioning metabolism—there's nothing magical or difficult about it. You just gotta. . . . .

EAT, BREATHE, AND MOVE.

LIVE

My husband and I are doing this together. I've lost a few inches, but he is doing so much better. We're eating the same foods and exercising together—why can't I lose weight as fast as he can?

Because you're not your husband, you have different bodies, probably different metabolic rates, different fitness levels, different everything.

Don't compare your success to his—you are much smarter, more wonderful, and more evolved than man could be—you're a woman!!!!!

For all you men out there getting ready to throw this book against the wall, that's a little joke. . . .

Your success is about YOU. Your fitness level, your goals, your physical considerations. To hell with everyone else's body but yours.

You will get lean, strong, and healthy if you eat, breathe, and move. So do it. Enjoy it, and monitor your success based only on your body. Believe me, it sure takes the pressure off and makes the whole process a lot easier.

Remember, Ginger Rogers did everything Fred Astaire did, but she did it backwards and in high heels.
—Faith Whittlesey

LIVE

My cholesterol is over 300. Will eating low-fat help lower it?

Yes and no.

First, you have to cut back on cholesterol (since cholesterol is the problem)—way, way, way back.

Then, you have to get your body well.

Healing arteries, increasing circulation, getting oxygen to every cell and muscle in your body, having your body strong and able to get rid of all the crap that's built up, and eliminating that cholesterol count of 300 is not going to happen if you are not well.

Sure, cutting back on fat and cholesterol is important—and not difficult to do at all. But lowering your body fat percentage, increasing strength, building your fitness level, and giving your body the oxygen it needs is just as important.

Get well, and live.

LIVE

My husband had a heart attack. Will this work for him?

The number one killer in our country is self-induced—and there is nothing more important for someone dealing with this disease than for him to stop with the saturated fat and cholesterol, get his body what it needs to start to repair his rotted arteries, give his body the enormous advantage of oxygen and strength by building lean muscle mass and cardio-conditioning.

But he can reverse it. Run to the store and get Dr. Dean Ornish's book, *Reversing Heart Disease*. Insist that your husband's doctor read it.

You have the control, and can take the choices that can save his life.

Yes, this definitely applies to your husband.

LIVE

I've had a cesarean. Will I ever have a flat stomach again?

If your doctor has indicated that the stuff hanging from the top of your section scar is anything other than fat, and told you that once you've had a section you can never regain muscle strength again . . . RUN FOR YOUR LIFE!

What's hanging from your stomach is fat, and yes, by all means, you can burn that off. The cut in your lower abs, or middle of your abdominal wall (depending on the kind of incision you had), does mend and the strength can be rebuilt in the muscle.

And let me ask you something: If you burn the fat, what's going to hang? If there isn't any fat there to hang, what you are going to have is a line—your scar—and a lean, strong, abdominal wall.

YES, YES, YES.

You *can* burn the fat off your stomach.

You *can* increase the strength of your abdominal wall.

YOU CAN HAVE A STRONG STOMACH AGAIN.

LIVE

When I quit smoking, I didn't start to eat more, but I gained weight. Why?

You see, it's more than the old oral fixation story that makes us gain weight when we quit smoking. You know what it is?

It's that smoking affects your body so dramatically, it makes the blood vessels to your heart, skin, brain, hands, and feet constrict. It decreases the blood flow to your sexual organs, and decreases your sense of taste, touch, and smell. It emits toxic gases inside the body, and it affects your metabolic rate— that is, speeds it up.

When you quit, you don't think your body is going to react or freak out at all? It does, and one of the ways it does may be by putting on a bit of weight. Why? Your metabolic rate doesn't have that nicotine kick. Your body has been bashed by nicotine and isn't functioning so well. Your blood vessels are constricted, blood is not flowing too well, and your sexual organs are screaming for help.

So, let's fight back. Start exercising—that increases your metabolism a hell of a lot better than nicotine does. Then, how about getting lean, strong, and healthy so your body comes back with flying colors?

I've done it—and it sure feels better than a cigarette.

LIVE

Since I've changed my eating habits, I seem to be going to the bathroom more often. Is this normal?

I'm assuming you're talking about going doody—you know, bowel movements? Well, I hope so, because this is a favorite subject of mine.

The moving of bowels thrills me because it is normal to move your bowels a couple of times a day, not once a week. When you eat high-quality, high-volume, less-processed foods, you become a bowel-moving machine—and it feels great.

Try eating a couple of bowls of brown rice instead of that laxative the next time you need to go. Change your diet just a bit and see what happens to your bowel movements. Bigger and better, I always say.

If moving your bowels is your body's wonderful way of eliminating waste, and you're not going to the bathroom, doesn't that worry you just a bit? Shouldn't we be just a little concerned about this, Doctor?

Your bowels and what's going into your mouth are connected. If you put processed, nutritionally depleted crap in, you don't get doody out. And if you put unprocessed, high-volume, high-quality, low-fat foods in, you won't believe what you get out.

There's nothing better than a great bowel movement, I always say . . . sometimes to the point of nausea, which I'm sure you are close to by now. . . .

LIVE

Is there some way to lose the weight faster? I have a wedding to attend in two months and I need to lose 60 pounds before I let anyone see me.

Don't go to the wedding. Lie. Say you've got the flu. You've probably lied for less reason than this wedding.

Do anything you need to do other than try to lose 60 pounds in two months, because the only way to do that is to starve. If the pressure of this wedding is going to make you diet, which is going to make you fatter and weaker, which is going to make your problem worse. . . .

THEN DON'T DO IT.

Don't go, and spend the next couple of months solving the problem.

Then the next time you walk into a wedding you'll walk in leaner than you've ever been.

Forget the 60 pounds, forget the two-month-I've-got-a-wedding-to-go-to time frame—and solve the problem.

No person is your friend who demands your silence or denies your right to grow.

—Alice Walker

LIVE

Why do some people get faster results than others?

Some people:
Put in more effort.
Eat less fat in their daily intake.
Have a greater commitment or discipline.
Want it more than others.

Some people:
Have less fat to burn so they look smaller faster than others.

Some people, some people, some people—
I don't care about SOME PEOPLE.

I just care about you, your fitness goal, your physical considerations, and your wellness.
Some people just seem to have it all, but you and I know that nobody has it all—we've all got something to deal with.
So think about you.
Your results.
Your body.

Let me listen to me and not to them.
Gertrude Stein

LIVE

What is the best way to figure out my body fat?

The best, probably, is being submerged in water—fat floats, you know. Submerging is probably the most accurate body fat measuring method.

However, and I say this with great conviction, if you take an inexpensive pair of calipers to your weight loss counselor, doctor, dietitian, or nutritionist and ask them to measure your body fat percentage, it's going to be close enough to give you a very good idea of how much body fat you have.

A point or two here or there—do you really care? Submerging, calipers, electronic devices—there are several options. I've always used calipers because I don't want to be dunked and anything electronic confuses the hell out of me. So for me and my clients, it's been calipers.

LIVE

I did my body fat with calipers and I'm off the chart. How can I measure my progress? Is it hopeless?

No. As a matter of fact, it's quite the opposite—so unbelievably hopeful that it makes no difference at all that you're off the body fat percentage chart. All it means is that you'll start measuring your success by getting *on* the chart and watching the number go down to whatever you want it to be.

Don't worry about it. All it means is that you are fat (and you knew that already!) and that you've got some fat to burn, just like the rest of the world.

Go, Go, Go. . . .

Feel good, get lean!

LIVE

*I can't stand myself. I'm so overweight I can't
even look in the mirror. What do I do?*

Don't look in the mirror.

You don't need to—you already know you're fat.

But stop disliking yourself—you are simply carrying too much body fat and walking around half dead.

We can fix that, so let's just get on with solving the
problem, instead of living with the symptoms.

Simple—it's time to change the way you look and
feel. You have to do what everyone else under the
sun has to do if you want to burn body fat, increase
lean muscle mass, build cardio-endurance.

You gotta . . . come on, guys, you know it—

EAT,

BREATHE,

MOVE.

*To keep a lamp burning, you have to keep putting
oil in it.*

—Mother Teresa

LIVE

Will it hurt me to take laxatives or will that help move the fat out of my body?

STOOOOOOOOOOOOOOPPPPPPPPPPPPPPPP.

Don't kill yourself because of bad information. Protect yourself by understanding what you're doing to your precious body. Laxatives to move fat out of the body? God, whoever told you that!

If eating a laxative or two moved fat out of the body, there wouldn't be a fat person left on the face of this earth, because we'd eat the fried whatever and then take a laxative, wait until it moved out of our bodies, and then do it again. But that ain't the way it happens.

Fat burns as fuel, and there's only one way to burn it.

MOVEMENT. Movement in oxygen. That's it. No other way.

Yes, yes, yes, taking laxatives to lose weight is extremely dangerous mentally and physically. Please stop. Don't hurt yourself.

LIVE

Do genetics play a part in weight gain?

Genetics has everything to do with everything.

But I'll tell you the truth here: 99% of us get fat because we eat too much high-fat food, and because we're not moving, we don't have enough lean muscle mass to stand up straight, and our bodies are not in good condition.

You may have inherited Aunt Mimi's bottom—but it may be Aunt Mimi's bottom covered in fat that you look at every day.

Once you get lean, it will still be Aunt Mimi's bottom, maybe wider than you'd like—but you can have a lean Aunt Mimi butt, or arms, or thighs.

We are all given different genetic compositions, thank goodness, but you can be short wide, broad-shouldered—and still be a lean, strong, and healthy short, wide, broad-shouldered person.

Whatever you've been given genetically can be as lean, strong, and healthy as you want it to be.

LIVE

My whole family is fat. Can I be lean?

Not if you live the way the whole family is living.

But cut back on your fat, increase the quality of the fuel you're eating, and start burning off the fat you've got stored on your hips and thighs—and sure you can.

You may have inherited a lifestyle that has to be changed a bit, but there's no reason you can't burn some fat, increase some strength, and change the way you look and feel.

I've been taking my two daughters out for brisk walks with me. We discuss good, better, and best foods. I don't want them to have the same rotten feeling about their bodies that I have had about mine.

—M.Y., Michigan

LIVE

How can I help my daughter? She has tried every diet on the market and nothing seems to work. I really want to help her lose weight before it kills her.

I wish I could give you an instant *Pocket Powter* answer to this question that would solve the problem. I can't, because as you know only too well, and anyone who has ever tried to help someone they love knows, you can't save someone from themselves. Everybody gets it at different times and for different reasons.

What I have tried very hard to do for people like your daughter is to get the information out there that really does work, that is easy to apply to her life, and that can, without a doubt, change the way she looks and feels forever.

It's available to her when she's ready to hear it, touch it, apply it to her life, and help herself.

Do it for yourself first—seeing you getting healthy, getting well and strong, is the best example you can give, and hopefully she will follow.

Good Luck!

LIVE

I really want to be healthy but I don't want to lose weight.

Bravo. Ladies, don't you just love people like this, no weight problem—don't need to lose a thing?????? WE HATE YOU!!!

Only kidding, just had to get that out.

Your question is a good one because there are a lot of people out there who don't have a weight problem—and again, WE HATE YOU—no, no, I'm back in control.

You are right. Health is important and even though you don't want to reduce body fat, you absolutely need to build lean muscle mass, increase cardio-endurance, and be strong and healthy. Eating, breathing, and moving applies to everyone, even those who don't need to reduce body fat.

Being healthy will increase the quality of your life, even the life of you naturally don't-need-to-lose-weight people. . . .

LIVE

I want to be healthy. Do I have to quit smoking?

All right, this is an interesting question.

The answer is obviously yes, but you can begin to get healthy *before* you quit smoking—if you want to.

You see, so many people wait until they quit to begin anything, but they don't quit and so they don't ever do anything to help give their bodies something to fight back with.

You can begin to move within your fitness level, even if you smoke. Cardiovascularly, you're gonna feel it, so remember, work at a low level of intensity.

You can begin to build lean muscle mass.

And you can sure as hell begin to cut way, way back on your daily fat intake.

There's no reason you can't begin to get healthy while you are working on quitting smoking. You may be amazed at how much getting leaner, stronger, and a little bit healthier can help you with quitting.

Start getting healthy now—and see what happens.

You just may quit.

LIVE

Will my stretch marks go away?

Never, ever, ever—but they sure as heck look a lot better when you're lean, strong, and healthy, and when you're running around in that bikini!

You know what else happens when you love the way you look and feel—you don't really care about those stretch marks quite so much!!!! I haven't thought about mine since I got into the grammar school sizes.

Today I bought new jeans in a size I've never worn before.

—P.A., Mississippi

LIVE

Does my metabolism slow down with age?

Yeah, it does.

But your metabolism also slows down with dieting.

It slows down because of a lack of exercise.

It slows down if you take certain medications.

It also slows down if you have the lean muscle mass of a jellyfish.

But your metabolism slowing down with age is not a given. Whoever said that after the age of 50 we should no longer function efficiently and with strength and vigor?

I know some 60-, 70-, and even some 85-year-olds who could knock the heck out of you and me, so—

Get well, and watch what happens to your metabolism.

When you cease to make a contribution, you cease to live.

—Eleanor Roosevelt

LIVE

When I reach my goal, what do I eat? How do I maintain my goal?

DANGER, WILL ROBINSON. DANGER, WILL ROBINSON! Diet, diet, diet mentality again.

That "maintenance" word.

Clear your brain of it because that diet mentality doesn't apply to this process.

You'll never reach your goal because your goal will keep changing as you get stronger and stronger, and more and more is possible. In the beginning my goal was to lose weight and look better than my ex-husband's girlfriend; now my goal is to begin weight lifting (strength training—don't worry, I'm not going to get that ugly muscly look anytime soon), finish my next book, go horseback riding with my kids, and learn tap dancing (me, can you believe it?).

My goals have changed since I've gotten fit because more is possible—so will yours.

You will maintain a lean, strong, and healthy lifestyle by eating, breathing, and moving according to your fitness level, your lifestyle, and your goals. This is easy to maintain—dieting isn't. Just enjoy being fit, enjoy your life, be well—and reach for the stars!

P.S. When you love the way you look and feel, you'll be eating just what you've been eating to get there—high-volume, high-quality, low-fat food.

LIVE

Can't too much of a good thing be bad?

Sounds like a line from an old musical. . . .

Yeah, I'm sure too much of anything is bad—but I'm not talking about too much.

I'm talking about anything:

Getting *any* oxygen, because we don't get enough.

Building *any* strength, because we are dying.

Reducing *any* fat, because it's crushing us.

Let's worry about the American public being too lean, too strong, and too healthy when that happens. We are nowhere near that happening.

Such a worry.

I'd welcome too much health and happiness. Wouldn't you?

Each day I ask myself if I'm feeling better and the answer is YES.

—L.L., Oregon

LIVE

I need someone to work with me daily and tell me what to do. Can you help me?

Yes.

That's why I'm writing this book.

That's why I wrote *Stop the Insanity*.

That's why I have audiotapes, videotapes, and everything else out on the market—so you get the information you need daily to change the way you look and feel.

The information's there—please use it, because it will change your life.

LIVE

How do I stay motivated to diet?

Dieting is hard to maintain.

No wonder we've had a problem with motivation—who could possibly stay motivated to starve?

You don't have a motivational problem. You are going to feel so good—that's what's going to keep you motivated. Your strength is going to come back after years of believing you'd never feel it again—that's going to motivate you! The motivation is in the process, and the process is fabulous.

Ask yourself these questions every day:

Do I feel better?
Do I have more energy?
Am I feeling stronger?
Am I shrinking?
Is it worth it?

If the answers are yes, keep going—keep going and don't ever look back.

Something inside clicked. I took a long, hard look at myself and what "I" wanted. The time has now come for me. I will make it "for me."
— B.L., Georgia

YOU
ASK, I
ANSWER

YOU ASK, I ANSWER . . .

This is not just my story.

This is the story of every single mom struggling to make ends meet, every woman who has a dream and wants to see it come true, every wife, every sister, every daughter, everyone of us who is thinking, planning, dreaming, and trying to get more control and choices back into her life.

As I've read through the letters, answered the calls, heard the concerns everywhere I've gone from the women who are changing their lives and getting lean, strong, and healthy, I've been asked a lot of personal questions, apart from the food, the oxygen, and the movement.

This program—developing it, making it happen, TV, books, radio—does have a personal side. I know you have questions about how it feels, what my plans are, about the ex-husband, and more—and I'll be glad to answer.

If you want to know about me, don't read the tabloids, ask me!

You asked—and I'm gonna answer.

YOU ASK, I ANSWER . . .

Do you ever get tired of talking about eating, breathing, and moving?

You know, I don't.

That surprises me, because I talk about it constantly.

There's so much to learn, so much new information, so many wonderful people who are beginning to understand—and so many different levels of understanding—that it doesn't get boring.

The more I read, the more I discuss with the real experts, the more I find out from you guys—the more I want to talk about it. Sharing and networking is loads of fun, and eating, breathing, and moving are so very important to all our lives that, what the heck, let's keep talking about it until everyone gets it—

Until we've learned all there is to know about it.

Then we'll talk about something else.

YOU ASK, I ANSWER . . .

Are you as fit as you want to be?

I'm fitter (more fit—which one is right?) than I ever thought I'd be.

Every time I reach a new fitness level, I am amazed at how capable and wonderful my body is, and how much more it can do.

My fitness goals change every time I get to a new level. So there's always a challenge, a new level to reach for, something to discover about what my body is capable of accomplishing.

However, the standard that doesn't change, and never will, is making sure that my foundation of wellness, my energy level, my peace of mind, my strength, and my body fat percentage are where I want them to be.

I told my husband the other day that I think I'll train for the New York City Marathon—talk about reaching for the stars! I've always hated jogging, and now the New York City Marathon?

Who knows?

What I *do* know is that now I have the option if I choose to take it.

THAT is the greatest joy.

YOU ASK, I ANSWER . . .

When you see someone who is fat and unfit, do you feel like you should say something?

When I see people who are physically hurting because they are so tired, or are so overfat, or don't seem to have any strength, sure, I wish that I could jump right in and start a conversation to let them know that they *can* change it if they just get the right information.

I have found myself in some restaurants wanting to pull up a chair next to perfect strangers and show them how they can order twice the food with one-third the fat—yeah, I've thought about it.

Many times I've driven by some of those diet centers in the shopping malls and wanted to sit in the parking lot and hand out copies of my book so that the people coming out won't become victims of the diet industry—and of the information they've just paid a fortune for. . . .

I admit it.

When I see people who are overfat, unfit, or hurting, I feel a burning desire to get them what they need to know in order to change their lives.

What do I do? I go back to the office, my hotel room, or home, and write about it, then get it published and get the information out there, hoping they'll pick it up, and it'll click.

YOU ASK, I ANSWER . . .

Is Stop the Insanity! only for fat people?

Stop the Insanity! is for anyone—

Anyone who can't walk up a flight of stairs without gasping for air. It doesn't matter what size dress you wear.

You are unfit.

Anyone who doesn't have the muscular strength to function. It doesn't matter how little you are.

You are unfit.

Anyone who is overfat—whether it's 10% overfat or 40% overfat.

You are unfit.

Overfat is overfat.

Unfit is unfit.

Also, anyone who is even thinking of dieting, and anyone who wants to look and feel better.

Male, female, young, old, fat, skinny . . .

Anyone who needs to *Stop the Insanity!* of starvation, deprivation, and being unfit . . .

Stop the Insanity! is for you.

Being overfat is only one of the symptoms of being unfit.

YOU ASK, I ANSWER . . .

How did you figure all this out?

Desperation. Passion. Anger.

A need to look and feel better.

And—after trying everything else, from starvation, deprivation, and obsession, to progesterone shots and lithium.

I tried it all—and it didn't work.

The pain that goes hand in hand with hating the way you look and feel, not having enough energy to live your life, and being unfit is something I will never forget.

That's how I got so determined to figure it out.

Then it involved tons and tons of reading, questioning, seminars, classes, discussions, and putting it all together. Breaking it all down—uncluttering all the crap, because there's a whole lot of it out there about getting well (as you well know)—and getting down to the foundation.

The foundation is wellness.

Then it took a lot of courage to start talking about it because I'm bald. I'm a housewife, and I was talking to the "experts."

They didn't like that much in the beginning. I think they're getting used to it now. If not, it's their problem, not mine and yours, because we deserve this information.

We deserve to be well.

YOU ASK, I ANSWER . . .

Was it hard for you to begin?

Yes, it was, because what I was trying to do wasn't talked about much.

It was considered nuts.

You have such an advantage. It's very hip to be low-fat now. High-volume eating is in vogue.

The information you need is here for you, so that your process will be a heck of a lot easier than mine was.

Organizing it and figuring it out was tough for me—but doing it was easy.

The process reinforces itself.

The energy you get from moving within your fitness level motivates and helps you move consistently, which gets you more energy to burn some fat, which drops dress sizes, which makes it exciting and encouraging, which motivates you to keep going . . . all the way.

The motivation comes from the process, not some outside magical source.

YOU ASK, I ANSWER . . .

How did you keep going?

By forcing my brain to look at what was, not what wasn't.

When I'd lost about 80 pounds, I was still the biggest woman in the exercise class. There were days when I'd hear the old tapes on the highest volume in my brain screaming, "What's the point? Look at your thighs. You'll never have good-looking, strong legs. Forget it—go home and eat."

Well, it took everything in my power to listen instead to the small, barely audible voice that was whispering, "But you feel better than you ever have before . . . five or six dress sizes are gone . . . and this is working without starvation or deprivation. . . . Keep going, don't stop, you'll get rid of the fat. . . . You can do it. . . . Don't look at everyone else's thighs, just think, keep going, and feeling good."

Well, Mr. Old-Tape-Loudmouth-Voice-of-Self-Destruction—have you had a good look at my legs lately?????????

YOU ASK, I ANSWER . . .

When did you first know you were going to succeed?

The first day I moved within my fitness level—and started to feel better.

The first time I walked for 30 minutes in oxygen. That small amount of energy was more than I'd had in years—and I knew then that I could do this.

Slowly, carefully, with food, I could do this.

Today, tomorrow, and the next day, I could do this. . . .

Step by step, literally, I knew I would get well.

YOU ASK, I ANSWER . . .

What's so different about* Stop the Insanity! *compared to all the other diets out there?

Everything you can imagine.

It proves that everything we've been taught is wrong—what do you think the people who've been "teaching" us felt about that in the beginning?

Then there's the level of respect for the American woman's intelligence that *Stop the Insanity!* insists on. I've been told by huge names in the industry that women would never use the fat formula because it's too complicated and they can't do math.

Can't do math? I can run a household, raise babies, do 10 times the work of you guys and get one-third the credit—and I can't do math?

Well, I said, WATCH US.

Watch us do the math, get well, change the way we look and feel, figure it out, network and support each other.

What women care about is the truth, and getting the information they need to change the way they look and feel forever.

Stop the Insanity! is different because it's the truth. No fluff, no muss, just the way it is. If you want to change your body—burn body fat, increase lean muscle mass, build cardio-endurance, and get your body looking and feeling good—there is only one way to do it.

YOU ASK, I ANSWER . . .

If what you're saying is the answer, why hasn't anybody said it before?

They have—and continue to say it.

Dr. Dean Ornish (*Eat More, Weigh Less*)—brilliant.

Dr. John McDougall (*The McDougall Plan*)—fabulous.

Covert Bailey (*Fit or Fat*)—wonderful.

Frances Moore Lappe (*Diet for a Small Planet*)—been saying it for 20 years.

Gary Null—talking, talking, talking.

Jane Brody—been writing big thick books for a long time.

The Goldbergs—great cooks, they know their foods.

Annemarie Colbin—really knows her stuff.

John Robbins—the best.

And so many more—check them out!

YOU ASK, I ANSWER . . .

Do you have a degree?

No.

I barely have a high school diploma. I dropped out of high school, then went back years later to get a degree. An associate degree in secretarial sciences, to be exact. (Years later, I say, Thank God for typing—who'd ever have thought that I'd be writing this?)

If I am an expert of any kind, I'm an expert through experience. It's a whole lot easier for me now to get to the real authorities and interview them, ask questions, and clear up confusion than it was in the beginning. When your book hits *The New York Times* bestseller list, all kinds of doors open.

However, from the beginning, I have been sure to check, double-check, question, and get the answer to the facts—and simply share my personal experiences with you.

In the Bible, it says that you are responsible before God for what you teach (I may be willing to challenge the so-called experts, but I ain't messin' with God). So call me a translator of information, expert by experience, an interpreter, or call me what I call myself: a housewife who figured it out.

YOU ASK, I ANSWER . . .

How can the diet industry get away with what they do?

I truly believe it's because we've allowed them to. I mean, think about this—we've run to them, thrown money by the billions at them, and begged them to keep ripping us off.

You can't only blame the criminal. If we choose to continue to be victims, then they'll continue to rip us off. We make it so easy for them.

Until recently, the diet industry hasn't been held accountable at all.

Now that someone is taking a look at what they do, and now that the American woman is getting so smart and demanding more, they're busted in a big way.

Not allowing ourselves to be taken advantage of, to remain victims, is a lesson that extends far beyond body image or health and fitness. That's something I've been learning more and more about every day—and something you and I will be talking about big time on *The Susan Powter Show*.

Think about it—and let me know what you think.

YOU ASK, I ANSWER . . .

I've seen your infomercial and wanted to know if that was a real seminar you were giving.

That first infomercial broke a lot of records—and one of them was filming a live seminar—unscripted.

Yep, that was for real, and that's what I do all over the country.

Next time you hear we are doing one in your town, come on down.

Whenever you fill an auditorium full of thousands of wonderful women, something interesting and special always happens.

I love doing the seminars, and will be coming to your town soon.

Watch the papers, listen to the radio, read your local newspaper—and join us.

YOU ASK, I ANSWER . . .

Why don't you build more studios?

Building studios is not the best way to get this information to as many women as possible. I could build a studio in every city and there'd still be millions of women who couldn't get to the classes every day.

But an exercise class that's out on video?

Lean, Strong, and Healthy is my class.

It's the class that I've taught for years.

It's a class that people at every fitness level can do—and change the way they look and feel.

I wanted to get this information to you in as many different ways as I could. Using different media—print, audio, video, TV, and radio to continue to network with and support women—is the best way I know to get this information out.

I've been working very, very hard in the last couple of years to do that.

If you want to read it—it's there to read.

Listen to it, put the audio in.

Exercise in the privacy of your own home—the videos are there for you.

Radio—count me in.

TV—it's coming to you every day. (You may very well find yourself in the audience participating and helping solve the problems!)

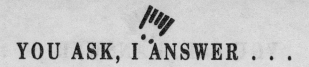

YOU ASK, I ANSWER . . .

What else are you going to do?

Whatever you need me to do.

More information, absolutely.

Discussion on TV for women, about women, and solving some of the problems that affect us all—that's definite.

Create more jobs for women. Doing that.

Feed the children—we are working on that right now.

My corporation is committed to the needs of the women and children of this country, and we are working in many different ways to solve some of their problems, making life a little easier, and create more opportunity for change in all of our lives.

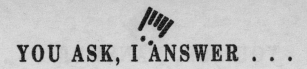

YOU ASK, I ANSWER . . .

Have you ever really eaten 32 baked potatoes?

Close to it.

No, only kidding.

Of course not. I don't know anybody who could eat 32 baked potatoes.

That was a fat-to-fat comparison—and a damn good one.

Stop the Insanity! is about eating a wide variety of high-volume, low-fat, high-quality food—not about eating 32 baked potatoes.

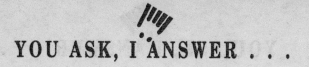

YOU ASK, I ANSWER . . .

What's your favorite food?

My favorite food is whatever I'm craving at the time.

If I've got a hankering for Chinese, then nothing is better than sitting down to that plate of Chinese food.

Mexican—don't ask!

Italian—unbelievable!

Sweet and salty combo just before my period—nothing could be better.

Ask me during one of my cravings, and I'll tell you it's whatever I'm heading for at the time.

YOU ASK, I ANSWER . . .

Do you ever eat fat?

Sure.

Sometimes by accident—the old restaurant chef who insists there's no oil in it, and after a couple of bites I realize there is, and send it back.

And sometimes quite deliberately.

The other day I went to the health food store and bought some (six, to be exact) eggless chemical-free, all-natural doughnuts and ATE THEM. Okay, not all six, only four. But there were 14 grams of fat in each doughnut. BLEAHHHHHHH, did I feel sick afterwards, but boy, were they good going down!

I'll tell you the enormous difference between eating that much fat now and when I was 260 pounds. At 260, that was breakfast, and there was more fat to come. Now, it's once every couple of months that I eat anything with that much fat in it.

Then, my body was functioning at a snail's pace; now, my body processes fat more efficiently.

Then, I was doing no exercise of any kind; now, I spent an hour on the treadmill that night when I got home, using up all that fat fuel.

So what's a few doughnuts now and then?

YOU ASK, I ANSWER . . .

When you pig out, what do you pig out on?

I love ice cream sandwiches.

Not the freezer high-fat junk—the Susan Powter specials that the kids and I devour.

You take your favorite low-fat ice cream and your favorite low-fat graham crackers and put tons of ice cream in the center, sandwiched between two graham crackers. . . . Smush it all down, lick the sides until you have a perfect square with moist sides, and eat it!

A big bowl of cereal is fun. Toast and jelly is a favorite. Low-fat potato chips go a long way. Ice cream floats—perfect on a hot summer afternoon. . . .

A million different pig-out favorites, but not eaten until after the high-quality meal—and never instead of the meal.

Our mothers were right—eat your meal first and then have a little snack if you want one. Then move, move, move—build that lean muscle mass, increase that cardio-endurance, and be fit.

YOU ASK, I ANSWER . . .

Is your hair naturally blond?

What are you—nuts?

There's nothing natural about my hair.

Every three days this natural, simple look needs to be cut and maintained—bleached, that is. It's the highest-maintenance hair you could ever imagine, but you know what? The minute I did it, I was thrilled, because I knew I'd found a haircut that I could live with and enjoy.

Lately I've been concerned about bleaching so much, because this bleach stuff has got to do something to my body. I'm thinking about changing—but not anytime soon, because I'm still enjoying this look.

When I don't like it anymore, I'll do something else.

But for now, this is it!

YOU ASK, I ANSWER . . .

Why do you cut your hair like that?

The hair!

My haircut was such an issue a couple of years ago that there wasn't an interview, a TV appearance, or a conversation with anyone that the hair question didn't dominate.

Thank goodness things have changed, because now my hair is old news and my program is what the media asks me about.

My hair truly is not a social statement, wasn't done for effect, and certainly wasn't thought about as a marketing or media tool—I would have been an idiot if I'd done this deliberately. In the beginning, this haircut made getting this message out feel like walking up a mountain in high heels.

I like my hair short. It looks softer bleached white than it does this short and dark brown (my natural color), and it works for me—that's why my hair is cut the way it is.

I hope that soon we are at the point that a woman's hair is not as much the issue as the person she is, the work she does, and what she stands for. I believe we'll get there sooner if women do what's best for them, and not be afraid to look the way they want to look.

YOU ASK, I ANSWER . . .

How old are you?

December 22, 1993—I turned 36 years old.

WOW—four years from 40, fourteen years from 50, and closer and closer to getting where I want to be:

Healthy, happy, evolved—the mother, wife, business woman, friend, and human being I am working really hard to be.

Age, time, and a lot of hard work get me closer to that goal.

YOU ASK, I ANSWER . . .

I read that you live with your ex-husband? Is that true?

The way these guys in the media word things makes all the difference in the world, doesn't it?

I don't live with my ex-husband.

We live very, very close together.

I have a duplex in Dallas, and he has an apartment downstairs, and I have an apartment upstairs. The kids have their mother and their father, and it works well for us.

This is not something that just happened.

Nic and I have worked very hard on developing a relationship that is fair to both of us, and gives the children what they deserve—both parents acting like adults.

Believe me when I tell you that it ain't easy going to counseling with your ex-husband, but every ounce of work that we've done has been worth it, because we have a healthy, happy wonderful family and my—oh, excuse, me, *our*—children are not the victims of a marriage that never should have been.

YOU ASK, I ANSWER . . .

Are you angry at your ex-husband?

No. I would never use a national platform to vent my anger at the father of my children. What you saw on the first infomercial and other TV shows is the truth.

When I say he walked out on me, am I angry—or am I just telling it like it was?

When I say he rode off on his white horse with his girlfriend on the back, is it male bashing—or the way it happened?

People who have read my book really understand and get a sense of what this whole thing is really about—and what it's about is the way it was, the way it is now, and the way it's going to be.

Nic is a very big part of my life. He is the father of the two most important people in the world to me. He's the man you could call a catalyst for this whole *Stop the Insanity!* thing. He is the person who has required me to put my ego, pride, and everything else I own aside so decisions could be made that are best for the kids, not the prince or me.

Have I *ever* been angry at my ex-husband—yes, angrier than you could imagine. But that was years ago, things have changed, and now there's a lot more than anger to talk about in our situation. . . .

I mean, after all, we live right next to each other.

YOU ASK, I ANSWER . . .

How much money have you made?

A lot more than I ever dreamed I'd make in my lifetime, but not quite as much as the newspapers and magazines say I have.

Let me tell you about making money. Anyone who says that being able to pay your electric bill without thinking doesn't make your life a whole lot easier is lying. It does.

But money can't make you happy when you are an unhappy sonofabitch, and I've met a lot of those. Money can't make you kind when you are hateful and unkind. Money doesn't help you wake up every day, grateful and happy to be alive, and money has nothing to do with walking around every day feeling like you've got everything.

My children, my family, friends, accomplishments, the women I've met, the goals and plans I have, and the work I put into me do that.

I had that without money—and I still have it.

YOU ASK, I ANSWER . . .

Are you happy?

I'm happier than I've ever been in my life.

The first 30 years were tough, very tough, but the next 30 years are going to be my design—and are going to be a heck of a lot better.

I have the strength to deal with whatever comes along.

I like what I am and am working hard on improving the weaknesses.

I adore my work.

The kids are healthy, brilliant, wonderful, and happy children—we made it together and love our family.

The marriage thing is going better this time around, and my husband and I work hard on making our relationship what we want it to be.

The women I've met during the last couple of years have enriched my life beyond my wildest dreams, and my life is good.

But I gotta say something here—my life is good because I work on it, and that's what I really enjoy about it.

I get out what I put in—and I put in a whole lot.

YOU ASK, I ANSWER . . .

What do your kids think of all this?

My children know only one thing:

A very short time ago, they had a mom who couldn't get through a day without feeling like she was going to die. A mom who didn't have the energy to participate in their lives. A mom who was very unhappy.

Now they have a mom who just went horseback riding in the mountains with them—and we had a great time.

They have a mom who is productive, happy, physically fit, and completely involved in their lives.

That's all they care about.

The rest is just what Mom does for a living.

YOU ASK, I ANSWER . . .

Are you ever afraid that you'll get fat again?

This is the first time in my life that I'm not living in fear of a lot of things.

Getting fat again isn't even a consideration in my life, because I know that unless I start eating tons of fat, stop moving, and let my body get physically unfit again, that's not going to happen.

So there's nothing to worry about.

If I had lost 133 pounds by dieting, I wouldn't have to worry—because I would have gained back the 133 pounds and more by now, and I'd be in worse shape (pardon the pun!) than I was back then.

GET WELL.

Then you'll never worry about it again.

There are plenty of other things to worry about, but getting fat isn't even something I think about anymore.

Thank God!

YOU ASK, I ANSWER . . .

Do you ever get tired?

Yeah.

After a 15-hour day—but that kind of tired isn't the same as the waking-up-tired kind of tired.

So tired you can't function.

Sick and tired.

Tired now is the kind of tired that feels great when you hit the bed.

Tired, as in well-deserved rest.

Tired, like needing to refill so you can go again tomorrow.

Tired, sure, but low energy, never.

Oxygen equals energy. Lean muscle mass equals energy. I've got plenty of all that, and as long as I do, I'll have energy.

That's why it's so easy to maintain, because the rewards of being fit are enormous. One of them is having energy.

YOU ASK, I ANSWER . . .

Do you ever get depressed?

It depresses me sometimes when I see how far women really haven't come—and how far we have to go before we can call ourselves equal.

When I have a fight with my husband, I really get depressed because I know how wonderful it should be—and when it isn't, it depresses me. You could throw a little angry in there as well.

Yes, I get depressed, but I don't stay that way for long.

I really try to find the solution to the problem, or get on with it if there isn't a solution.

Taking a couple of deep breaths, going for a walk, spending time with my children—there are a lot of tools I use to work through situations that are depressing.

But getting on with it is always the best solution. I mean, why sit in it?

YOU ASK, I ANSWER . . .

***Don't you think life is too short to worry
about all this stuff?***

Life is too short not to worry about this stuff.

Nobody knows when the big one is coming—whatever the big one is—but while you're here, whether it's a couple of years or a hundred, you may as well live a high-quality, good life.

I mean, what's the point if you're miserable?

Don't have any energy?

Sick and tired all the time and feeling like crap?

It doesn't matter how short or long your life is—make it all that it can be and get on with living, because living is big fun.

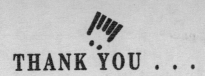

THANK YOU . . .

for sending me your questions and comments. Networking and supporting each other is the only way we are going to "Stop the Insanity."

Send me your low-fat recipes, your low-fat lifestyle suggestions, tips, comments, transition stories. Talk to me about the husband, the kids, the job—your life.

I'd love to hear from you and share information with all the wonderful women who are changing the way they look and feel forever.

Be well,

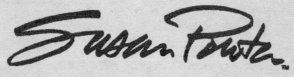

Please send all information to:

Susan Powter Corporation
P.O. Box 803331
Dallas, TX 75380

Or call 1-800-94-SUSAN
or -78726